THE PICTURE BOOK OF
FLOWERS

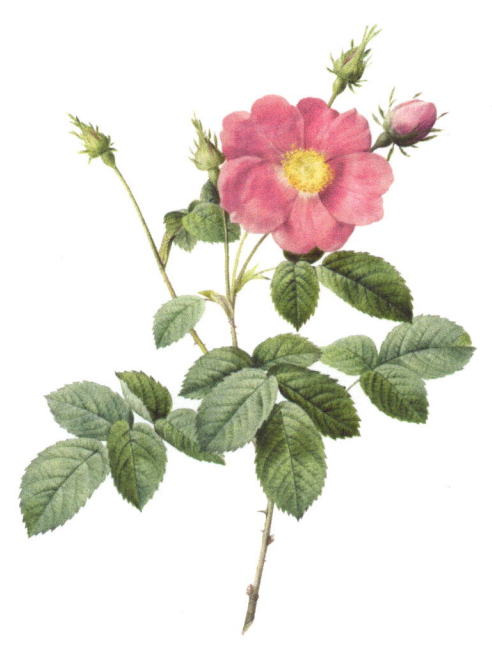

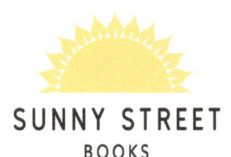

SUNNY STREET
BOOKS

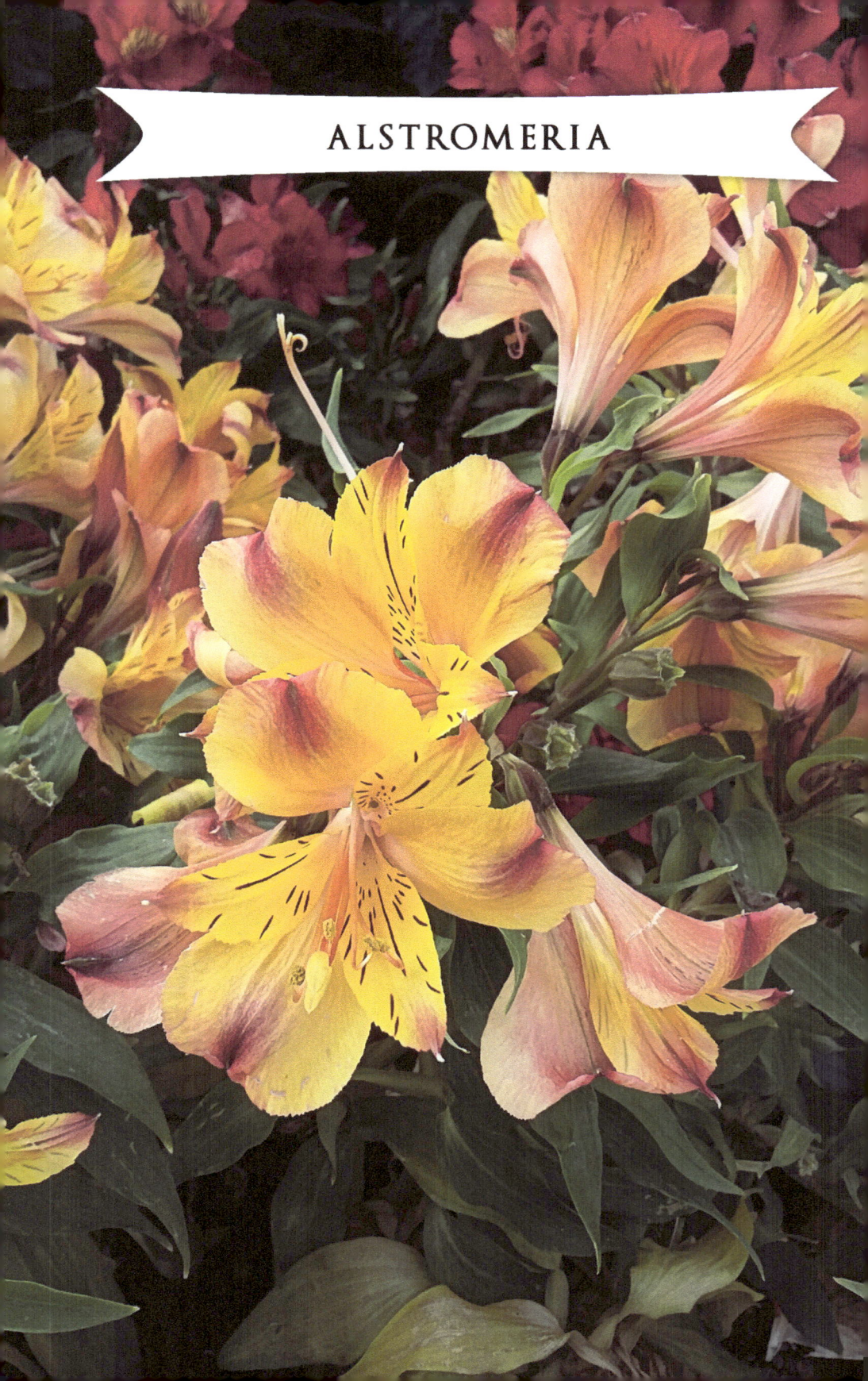

ALSTROMERIA

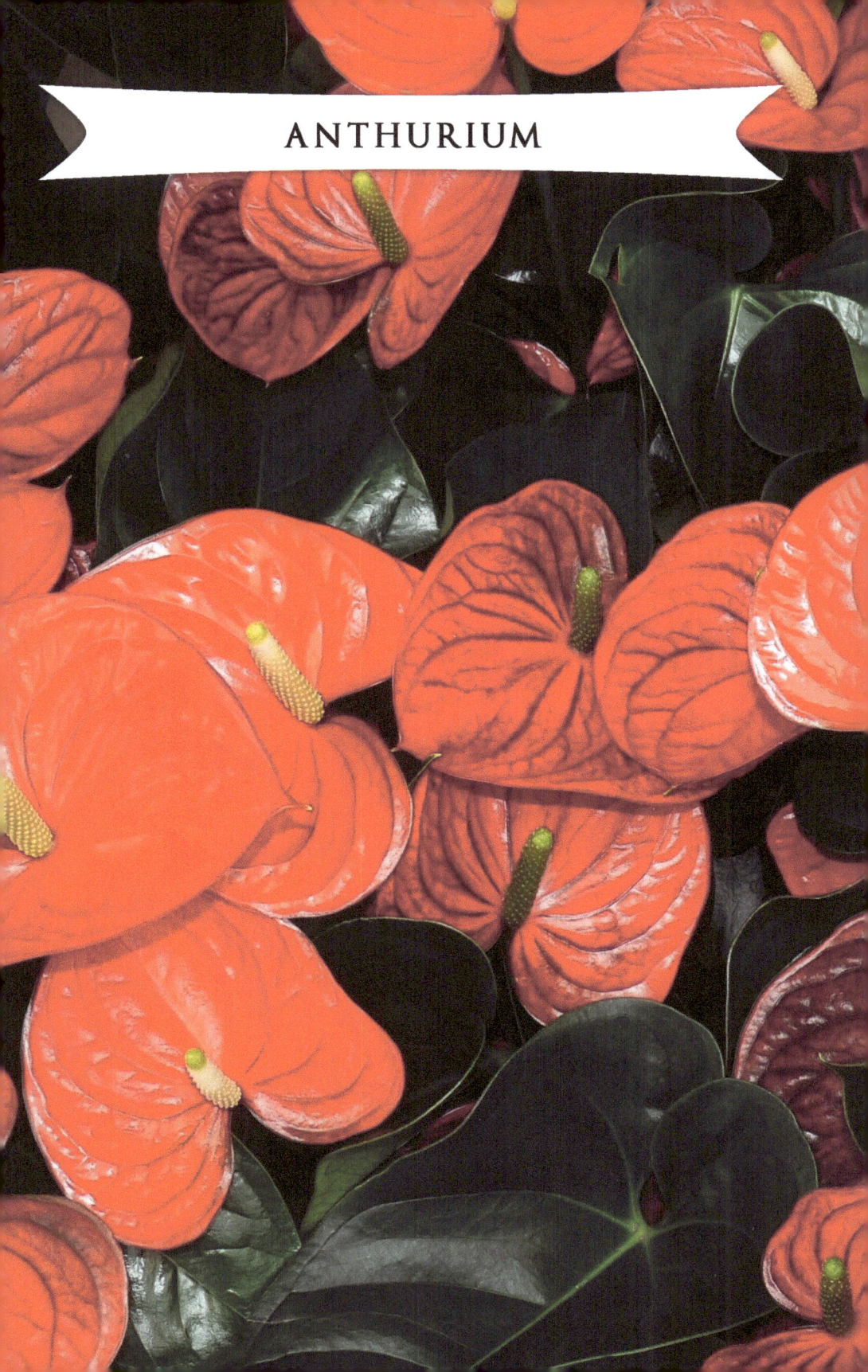

ANTHURIUM

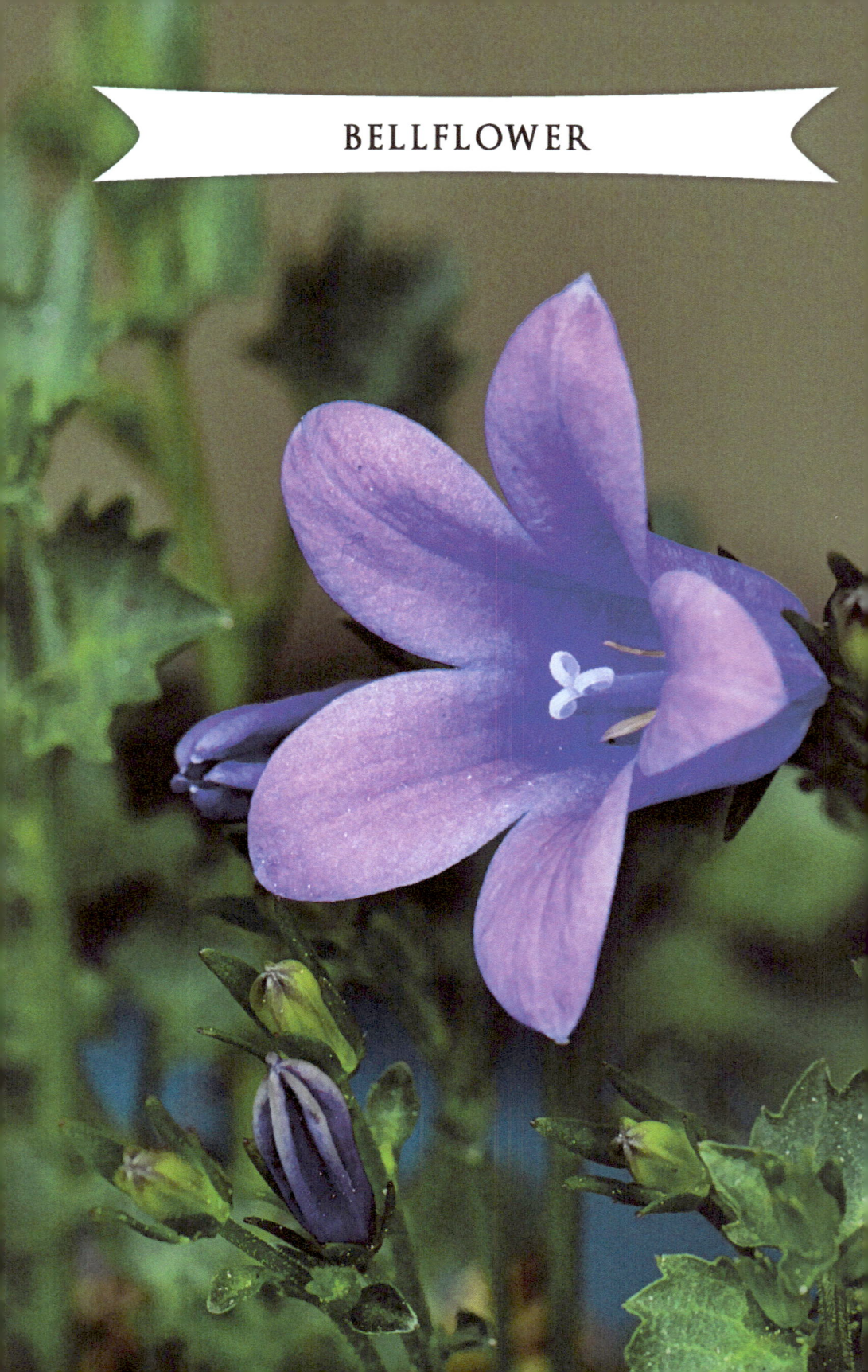

BELLFLOWER

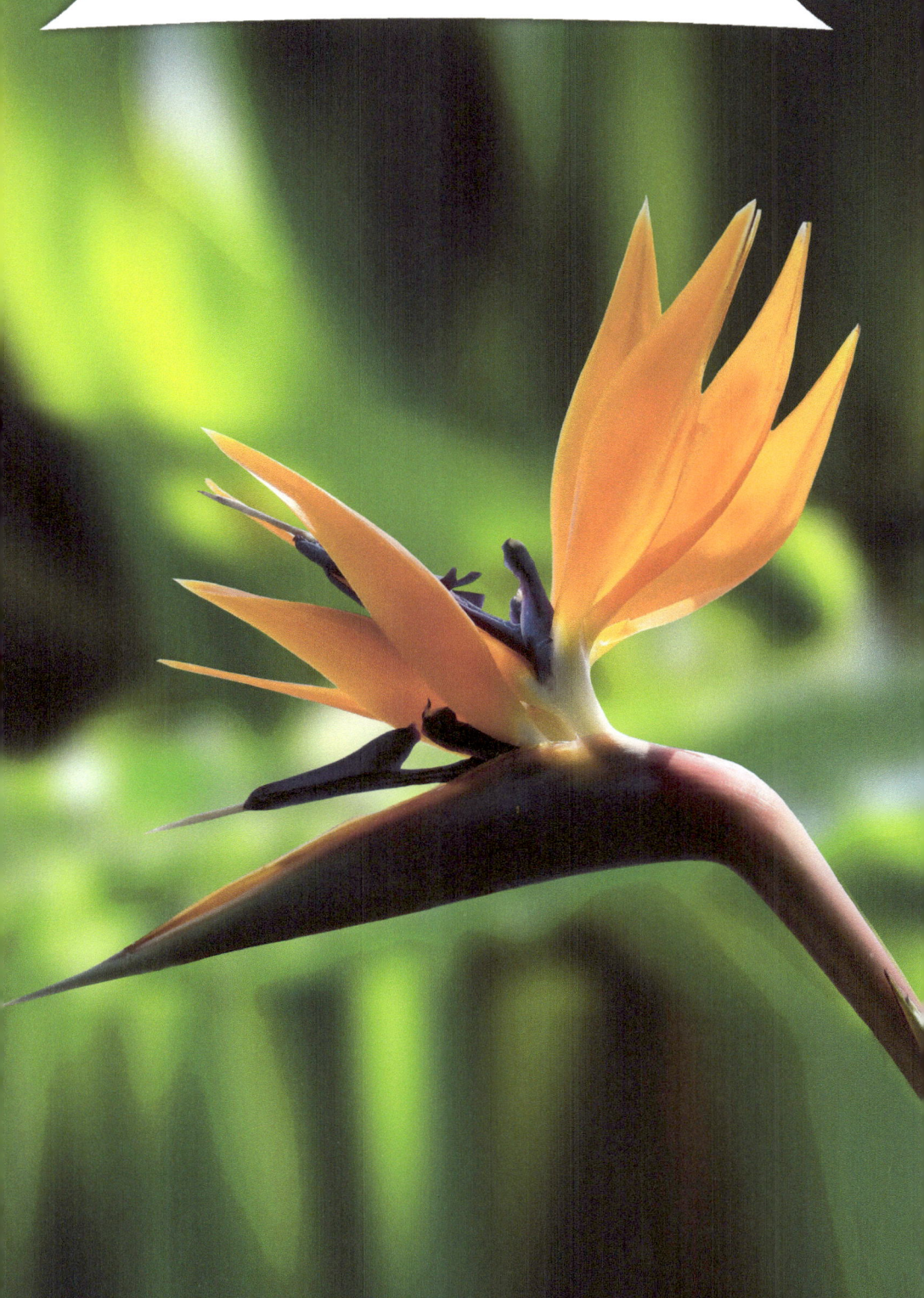

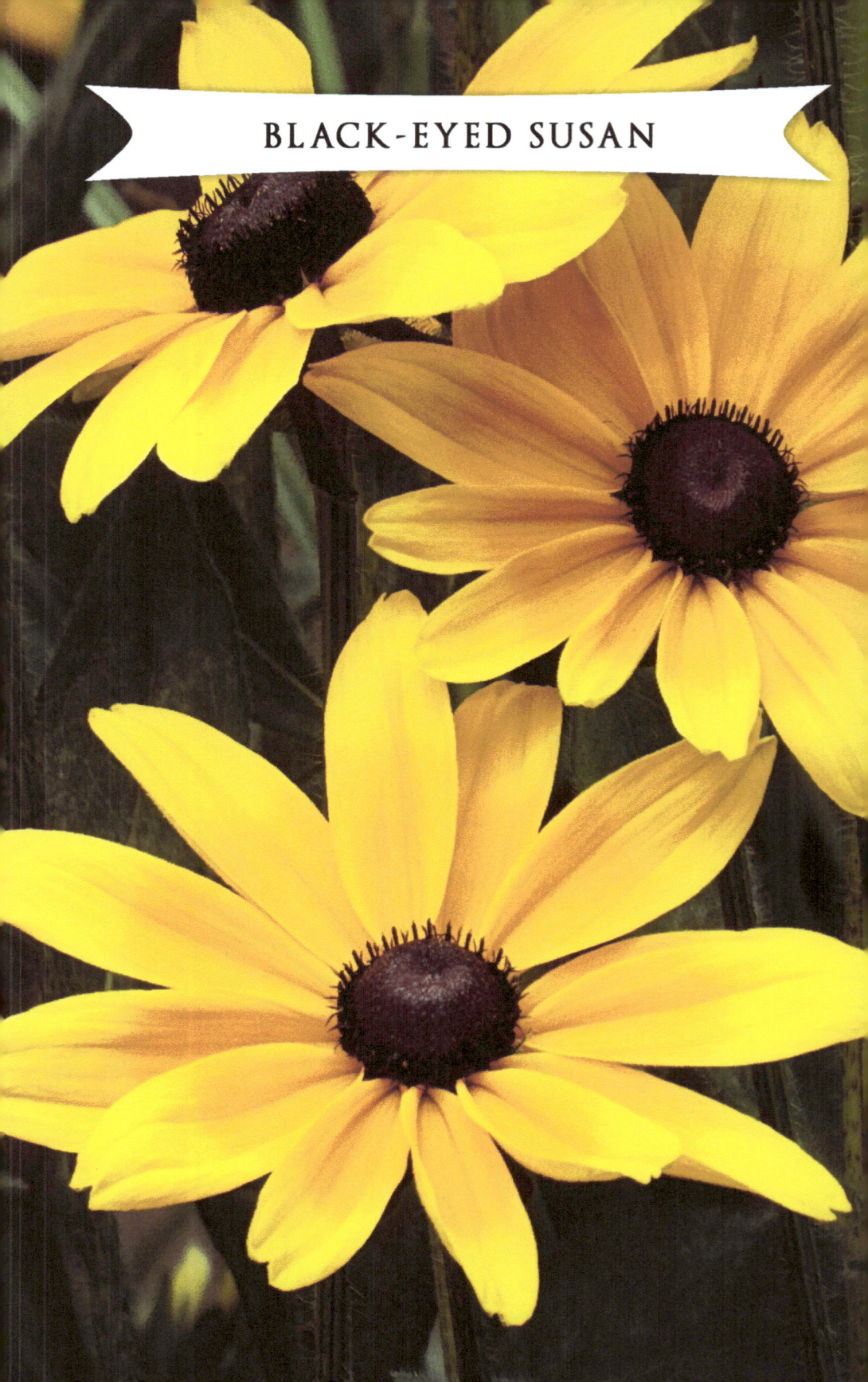

BLACK-EYED SUSAN

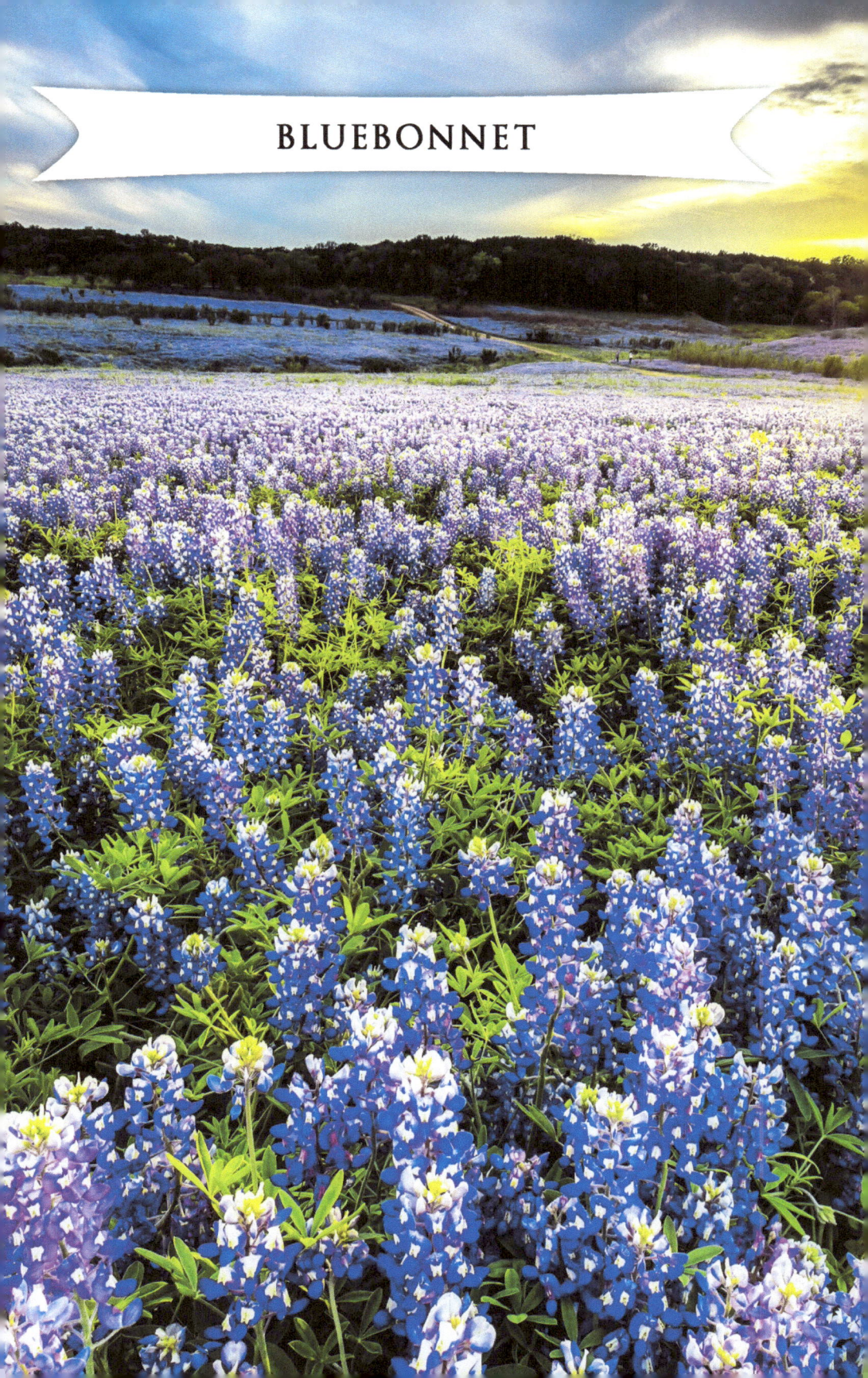

BLUEBONNET

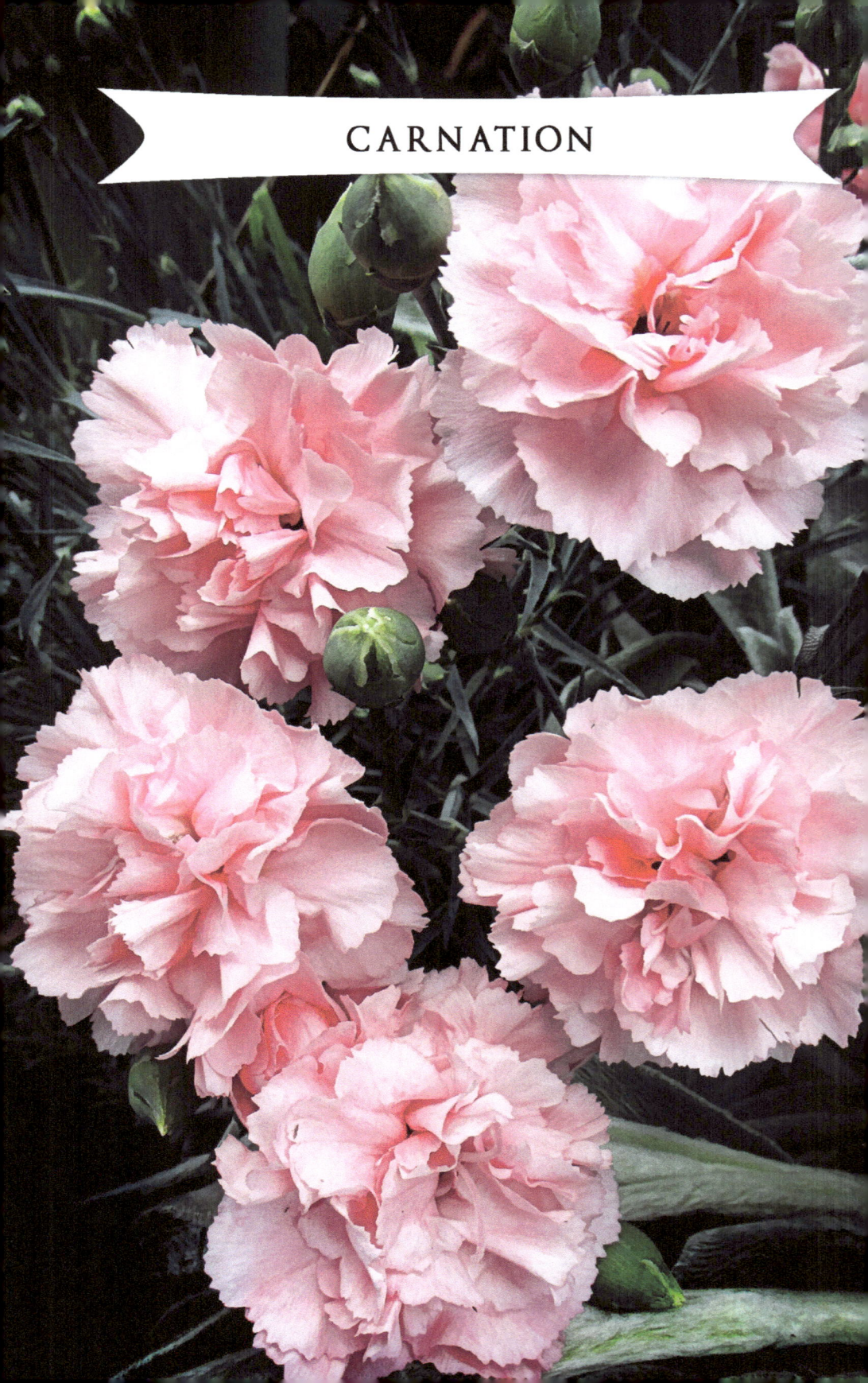

CARNATION

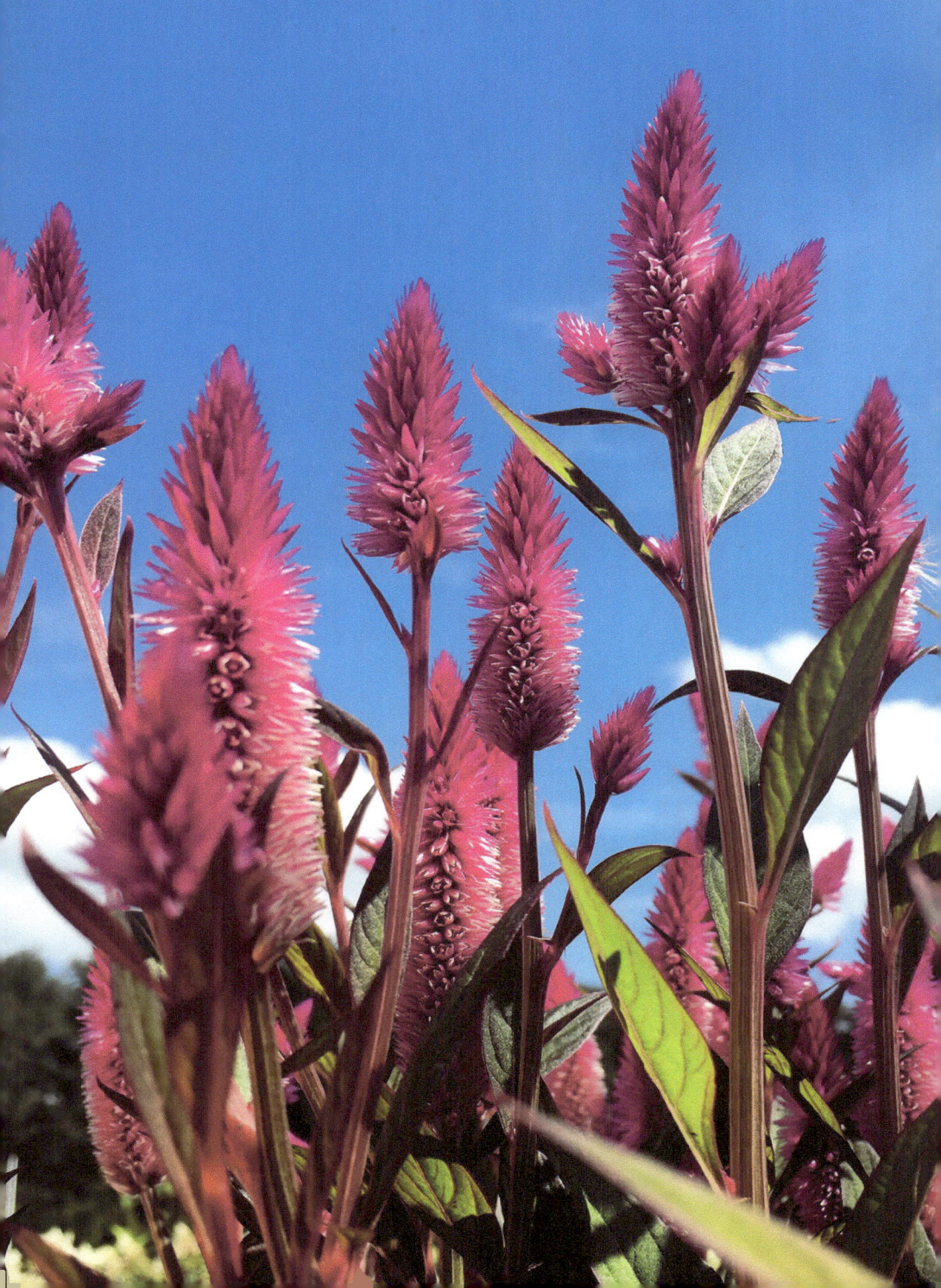

CELOSIA

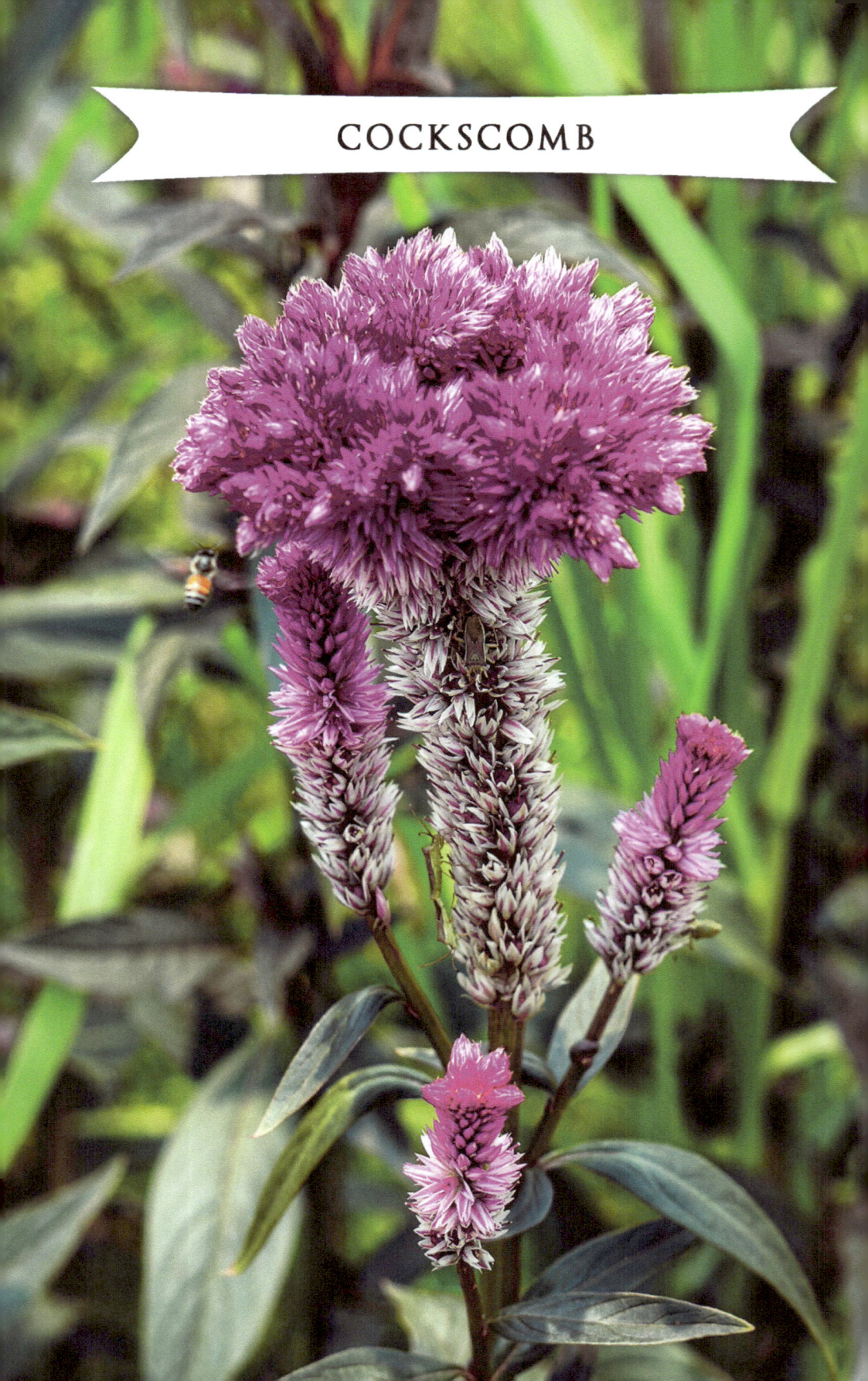

COSMOS

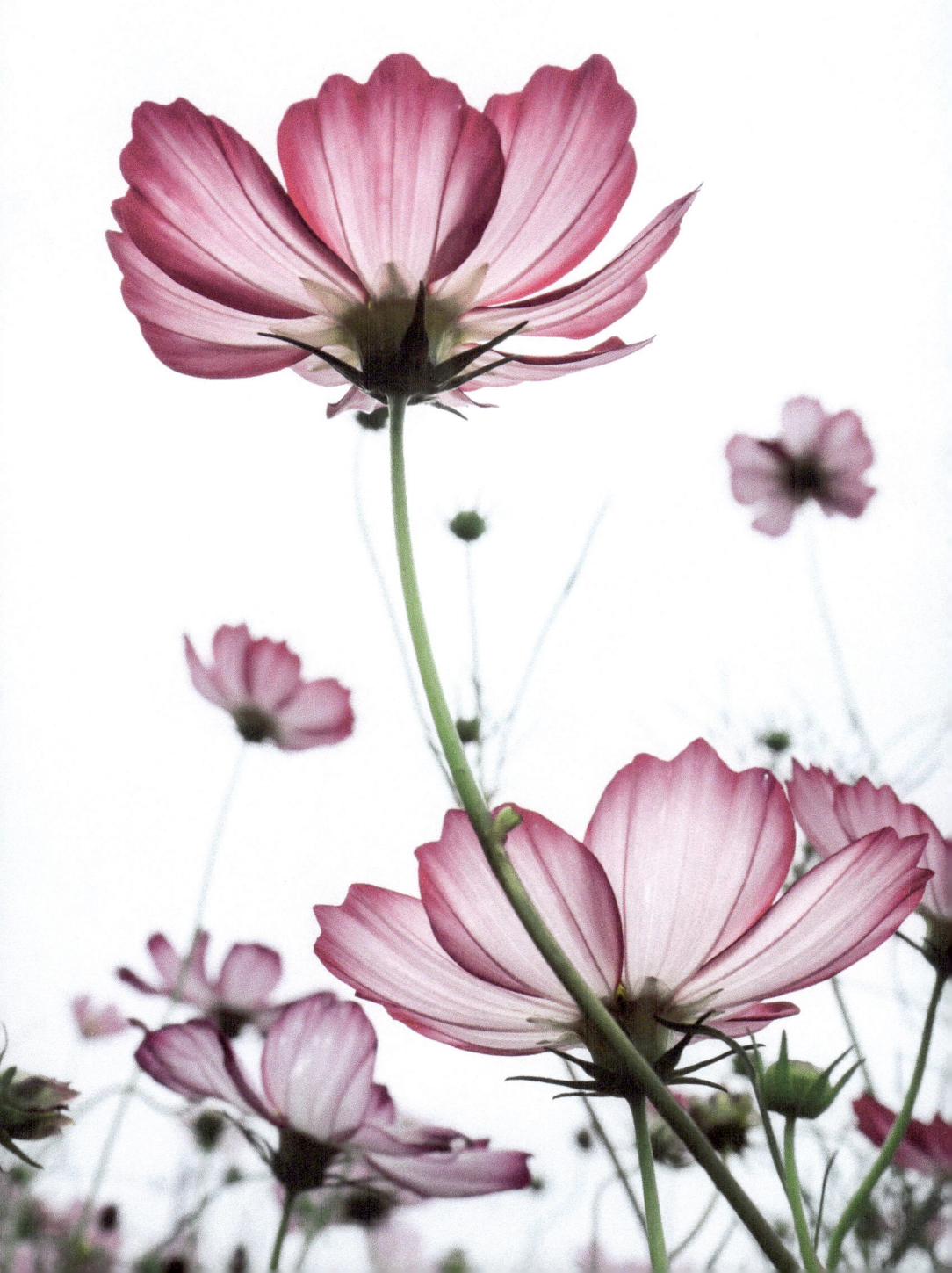

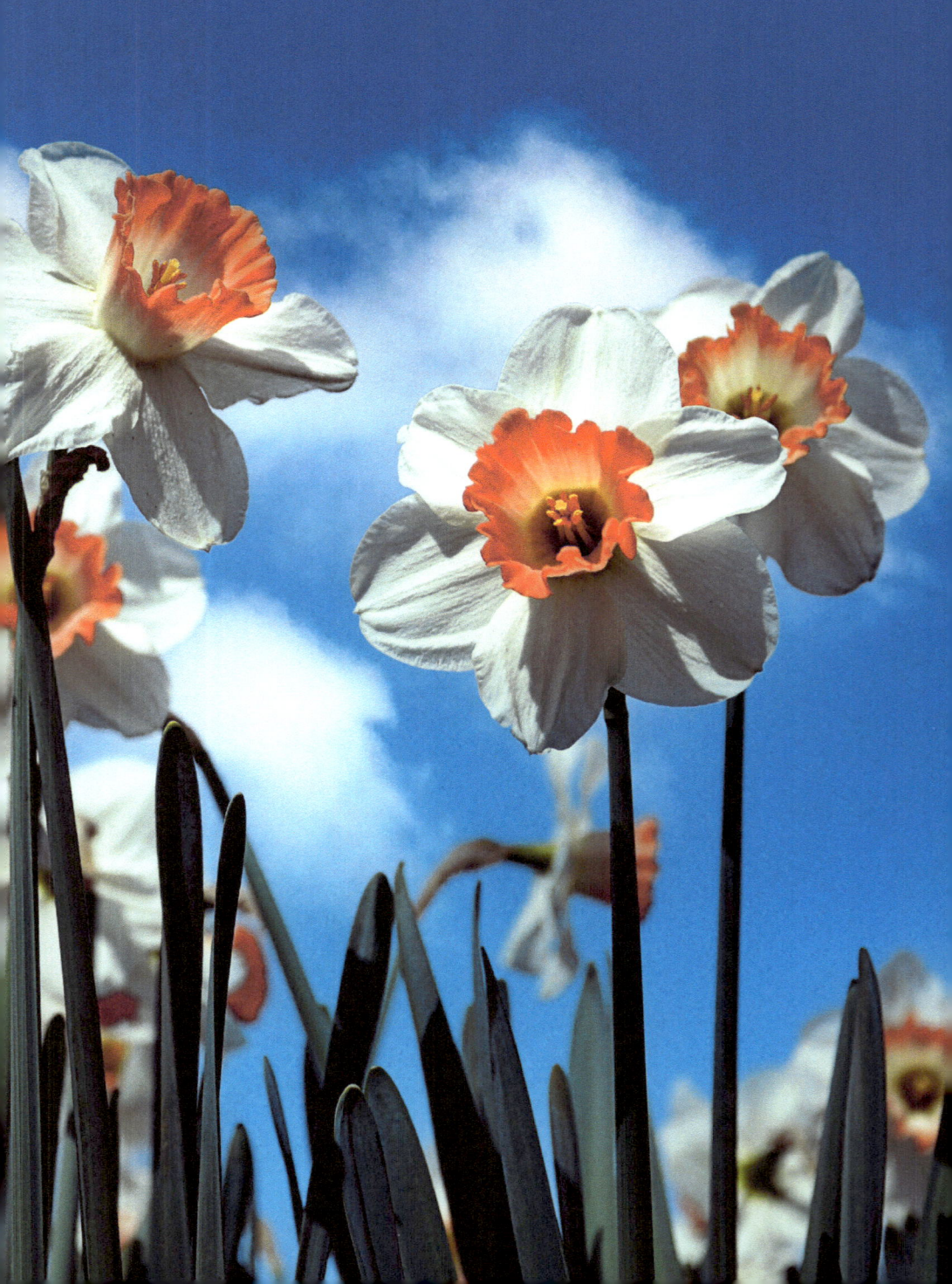

DAFFODIL

DAISY

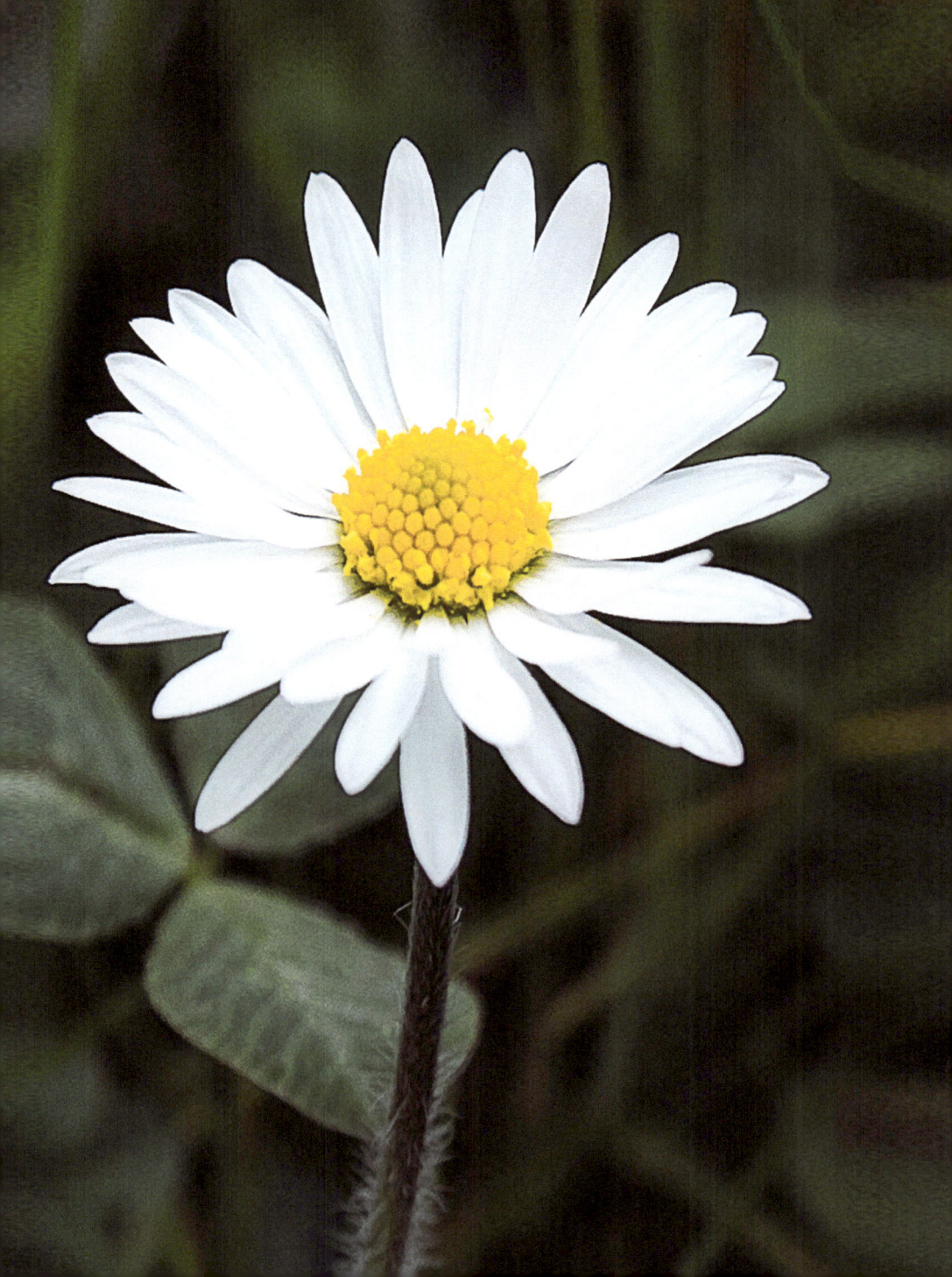

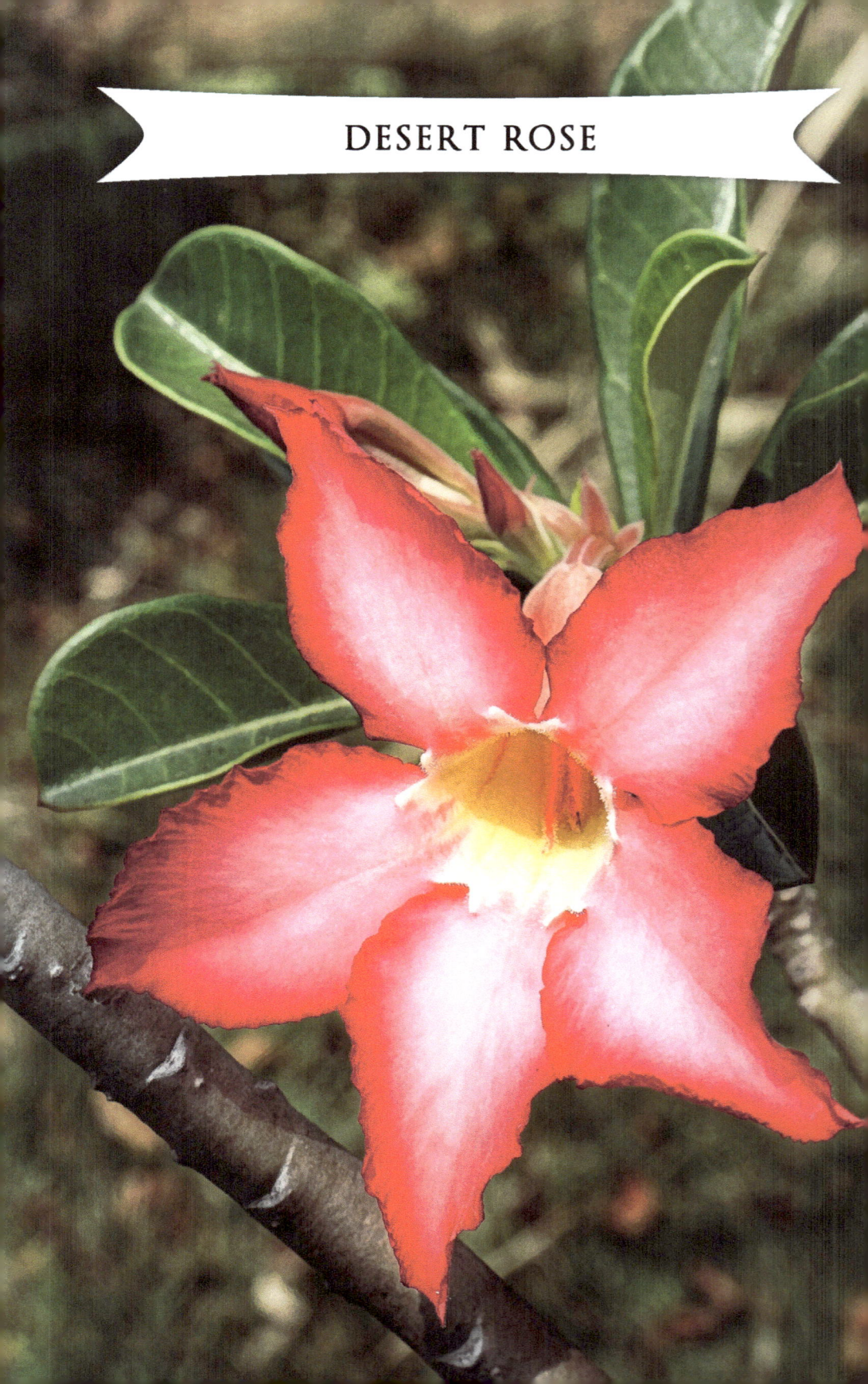

DESERT ROSE

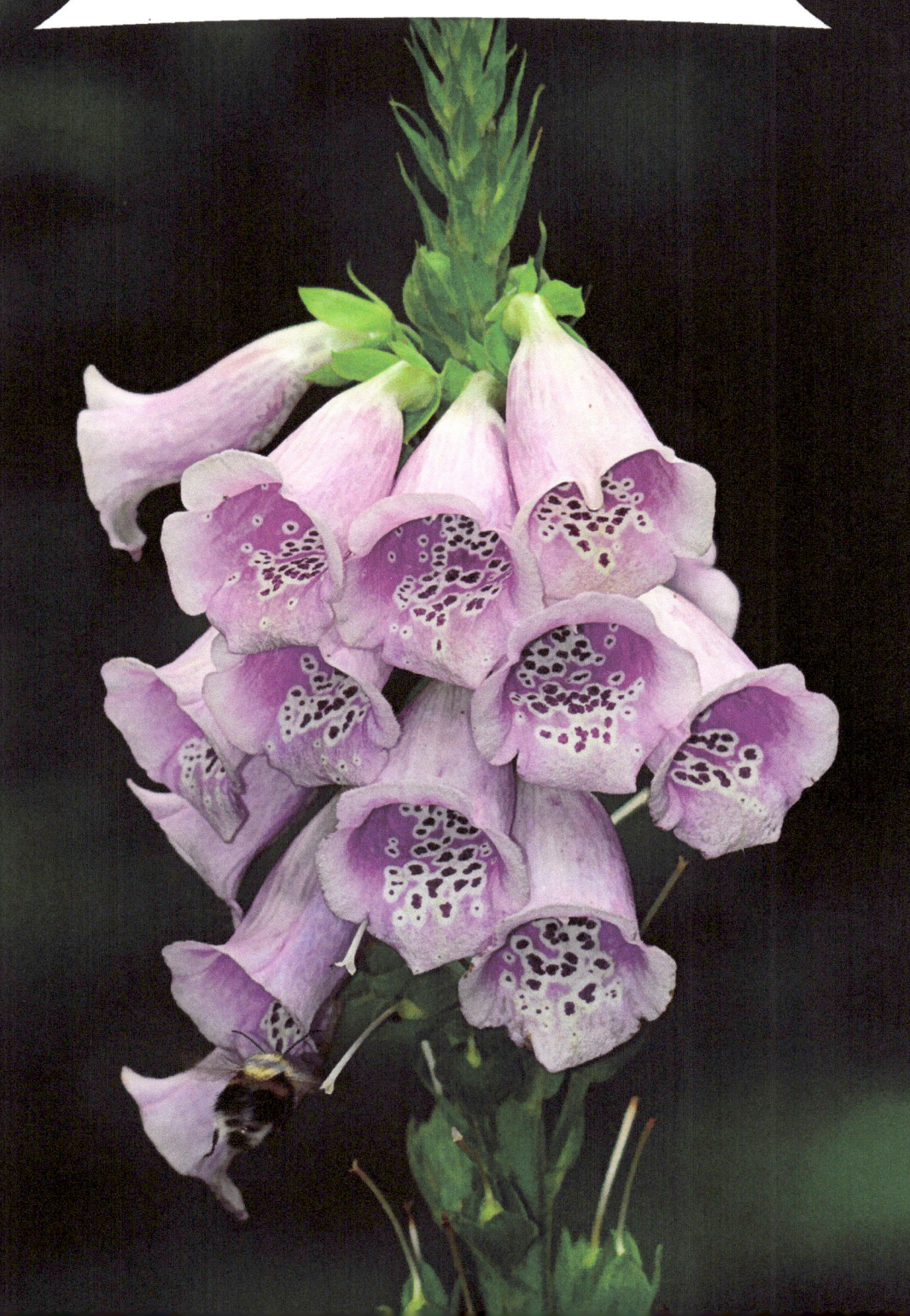

FOXGLOVE

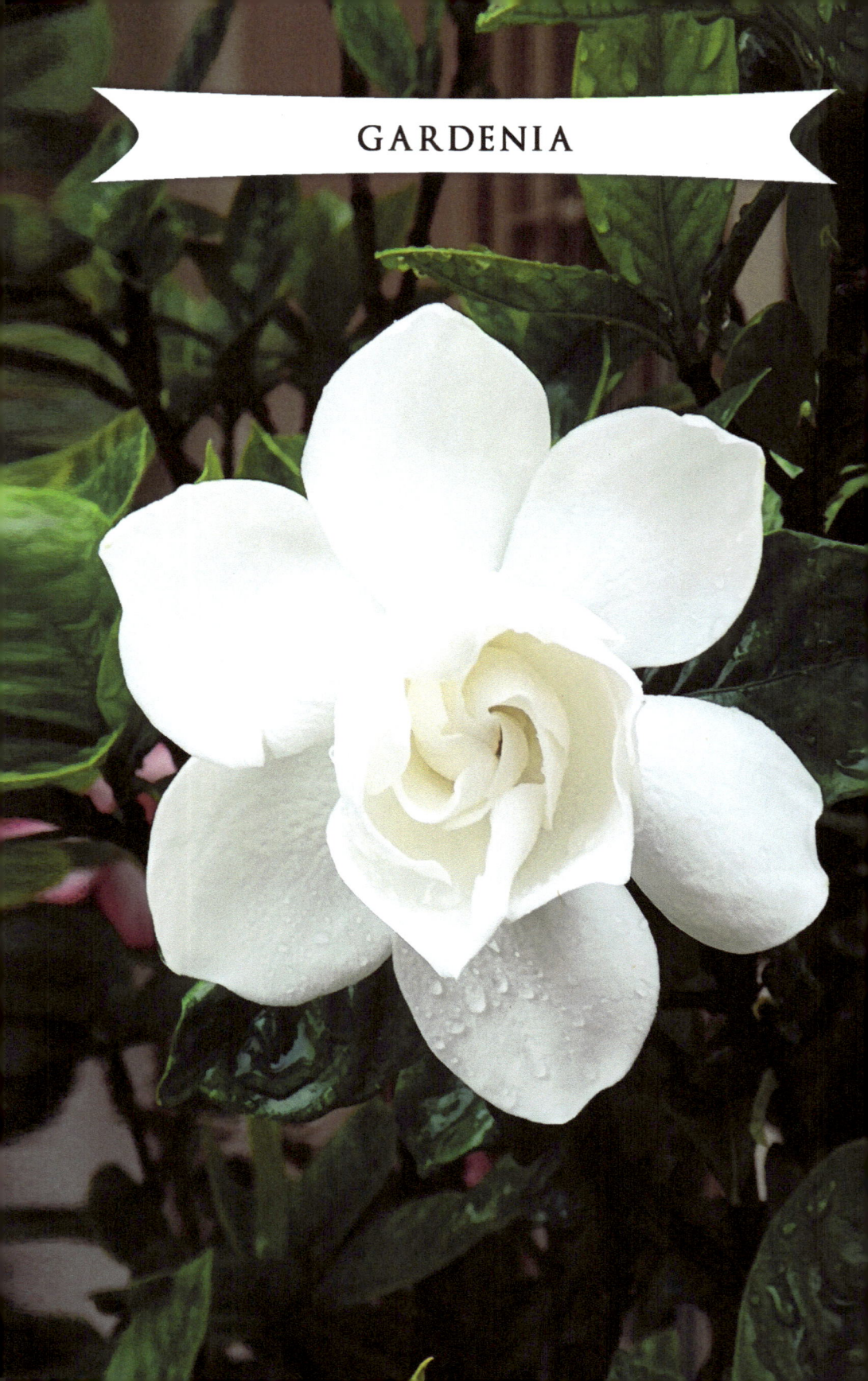

GARDENIA

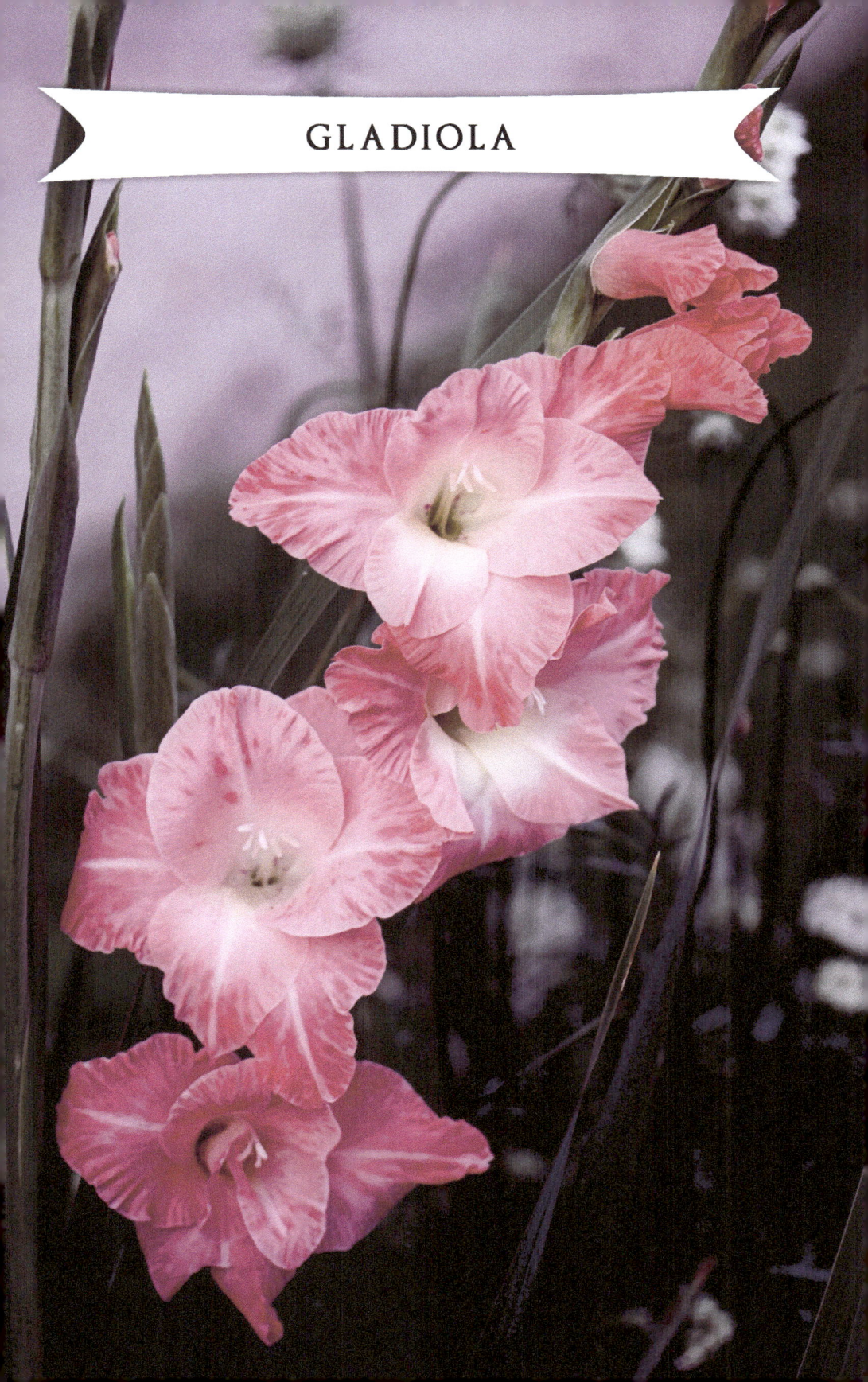

GLADIOLA

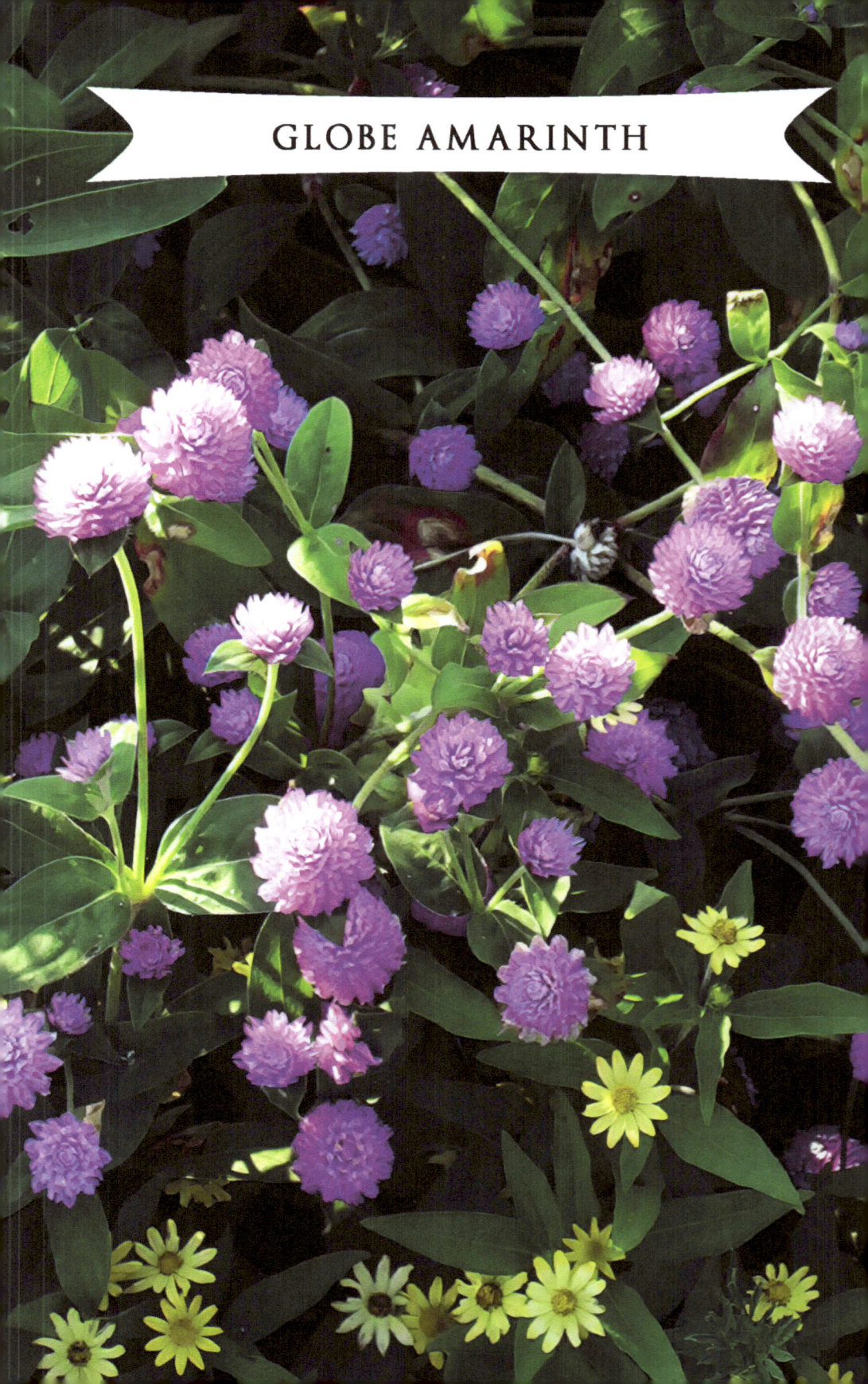

GLOBE AMARINTH

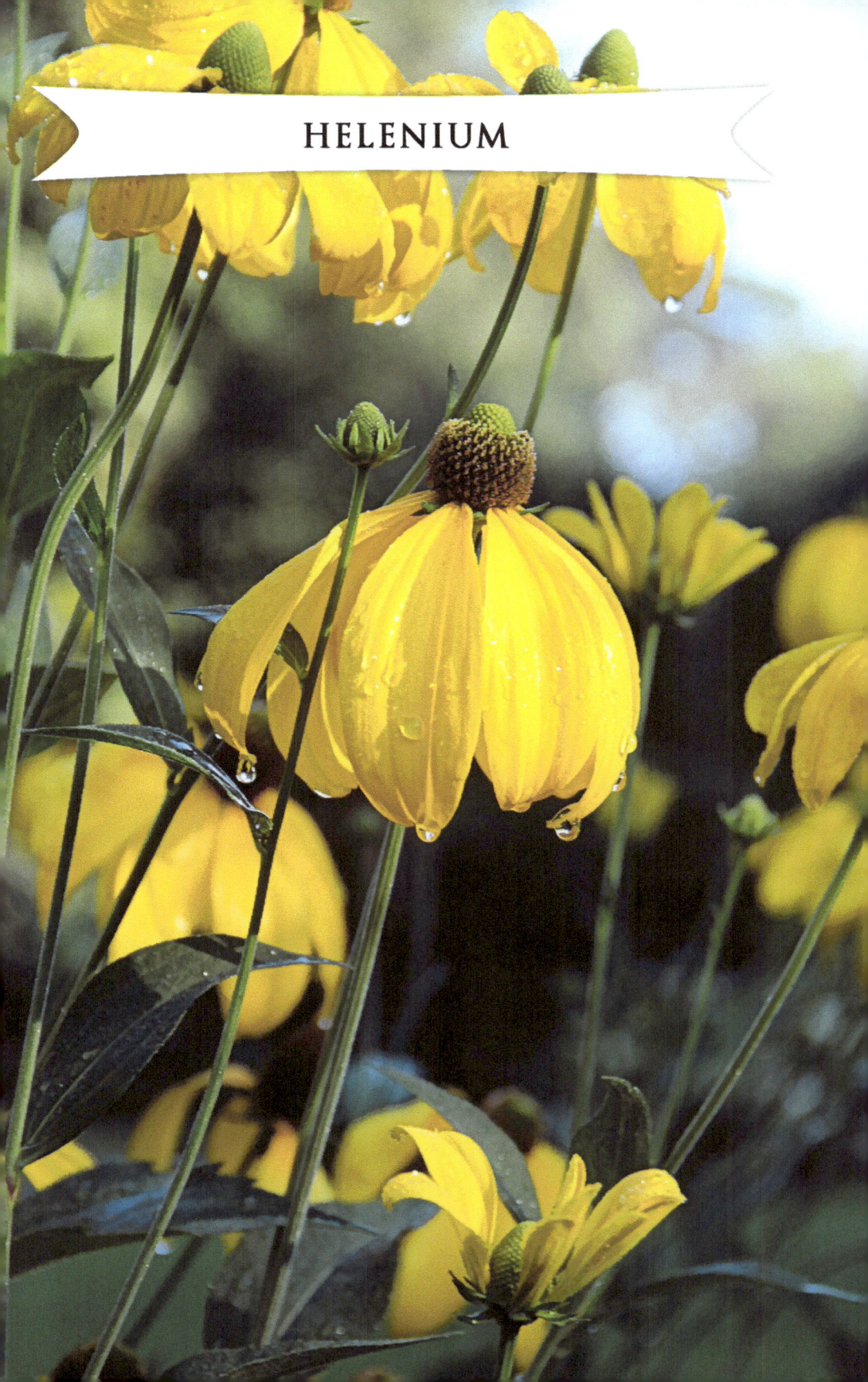

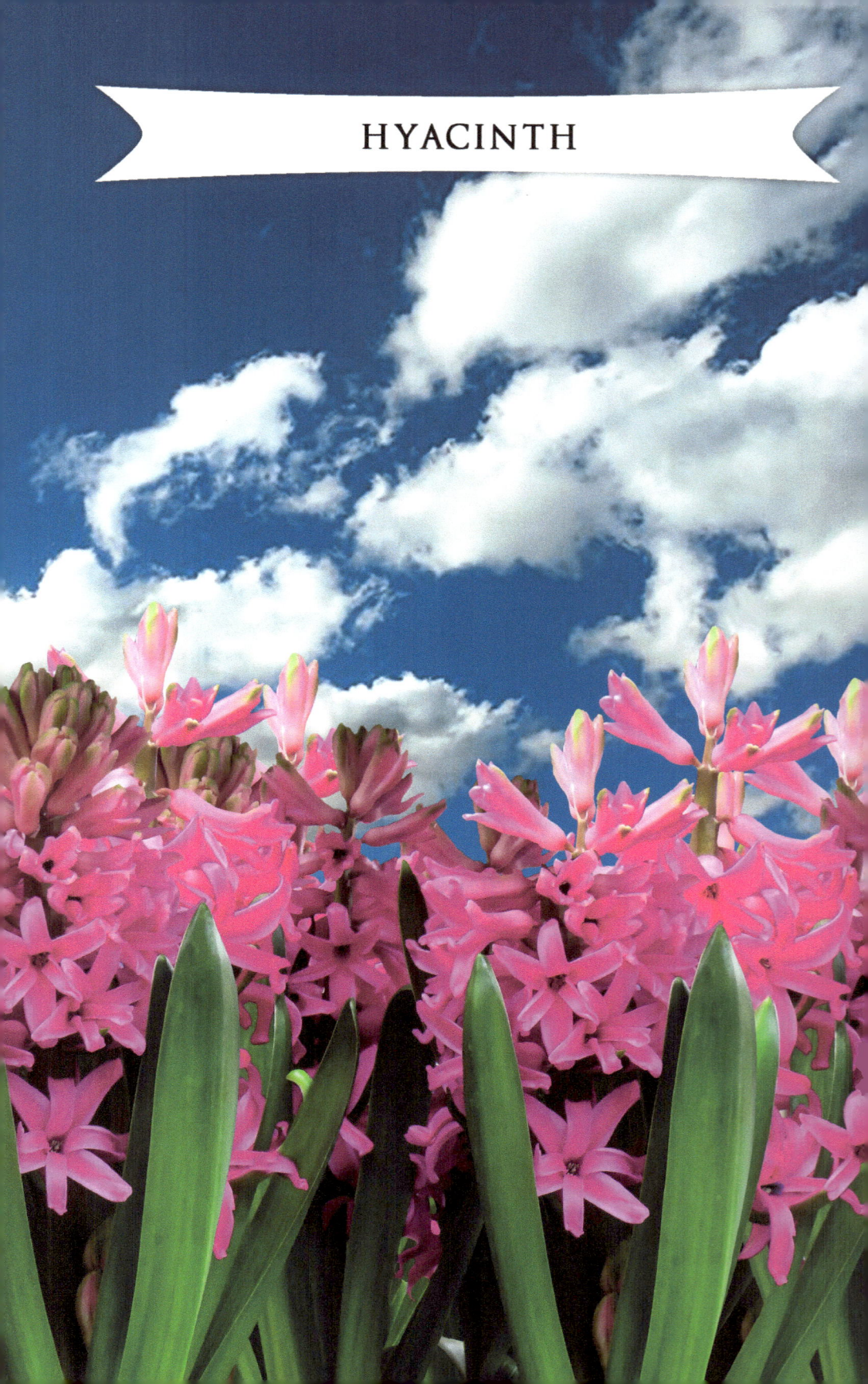

HYACINTH

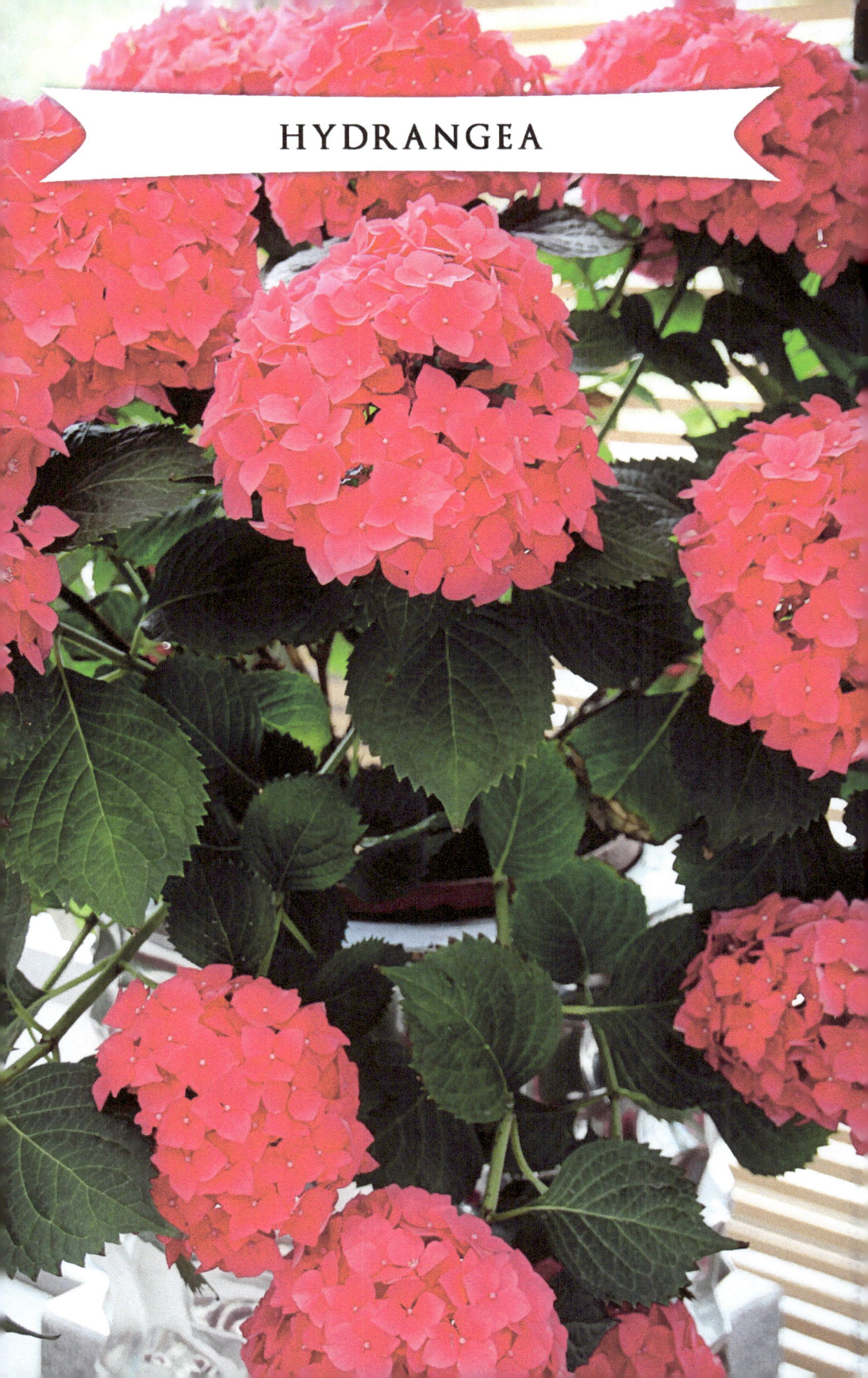

HYDRANGEA

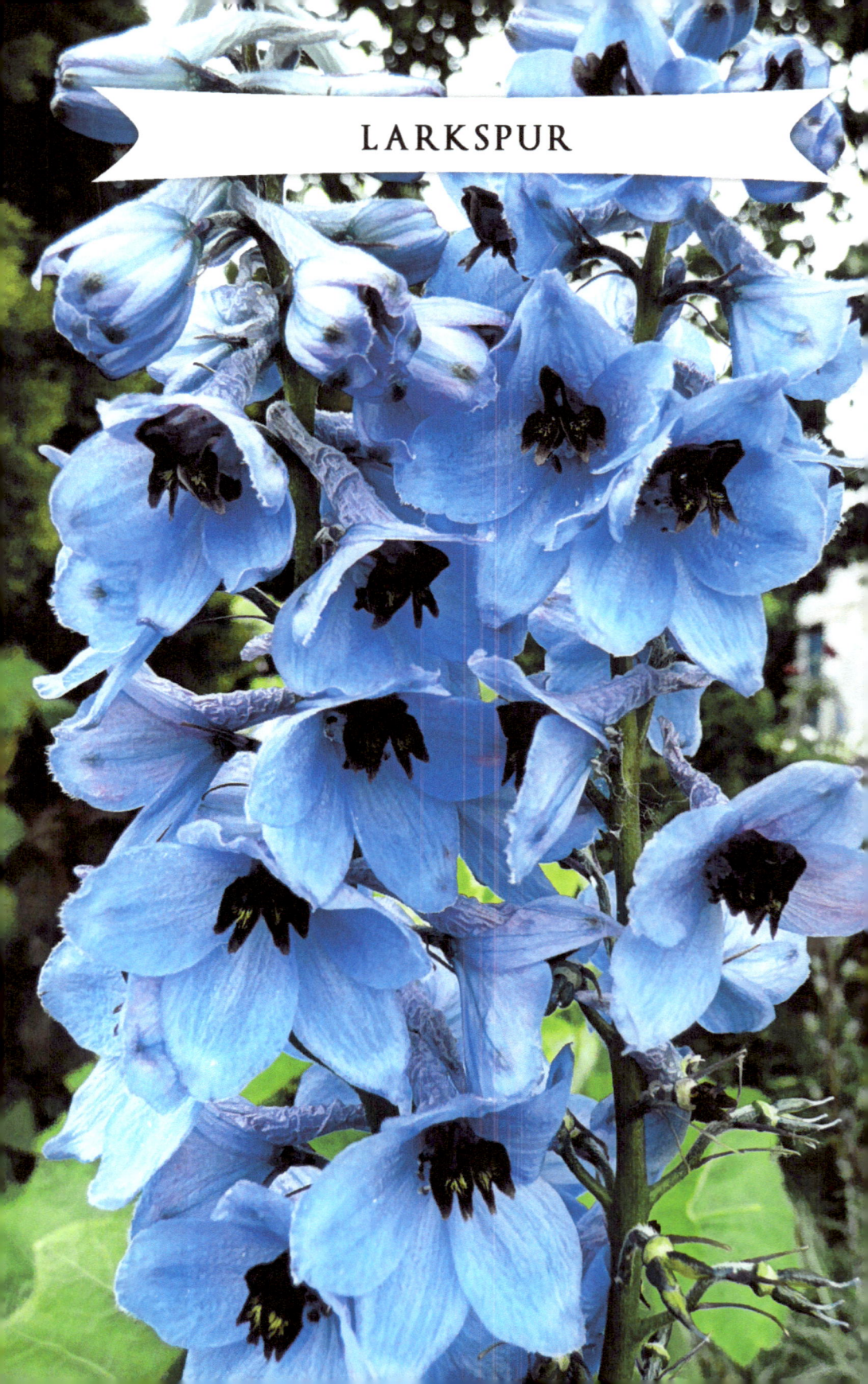

LARKSPUR

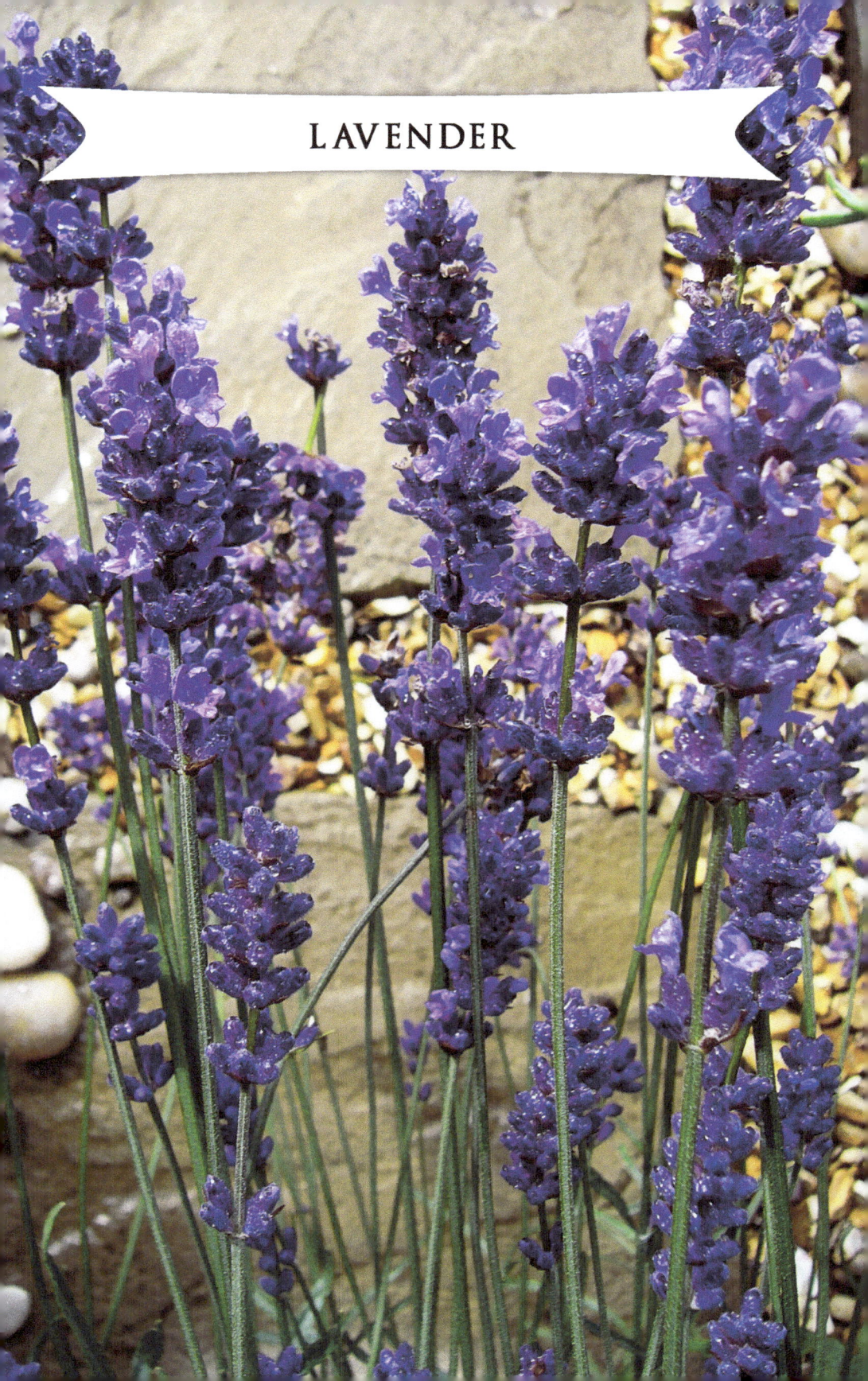

LAVENDER

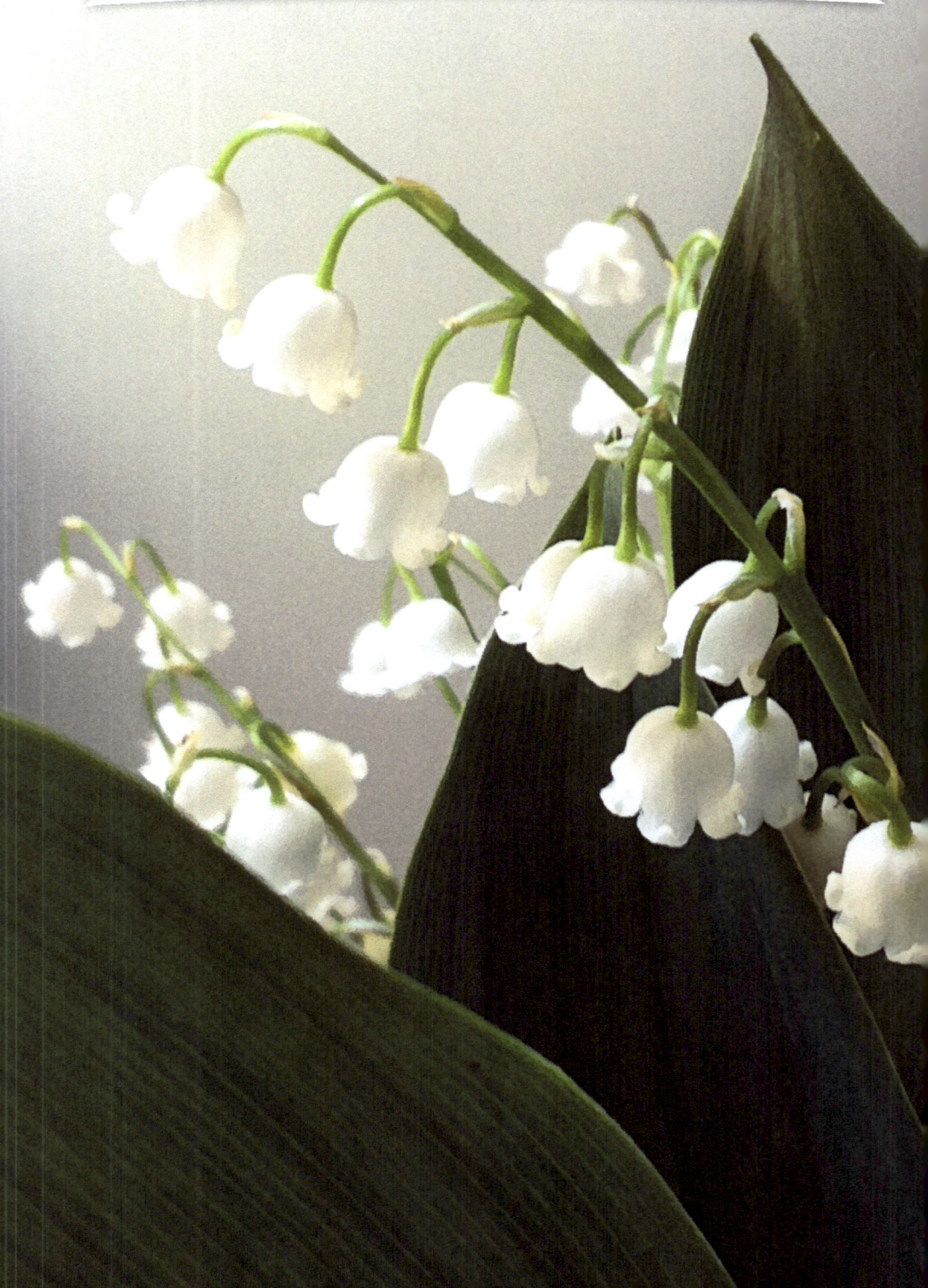

LOTUS

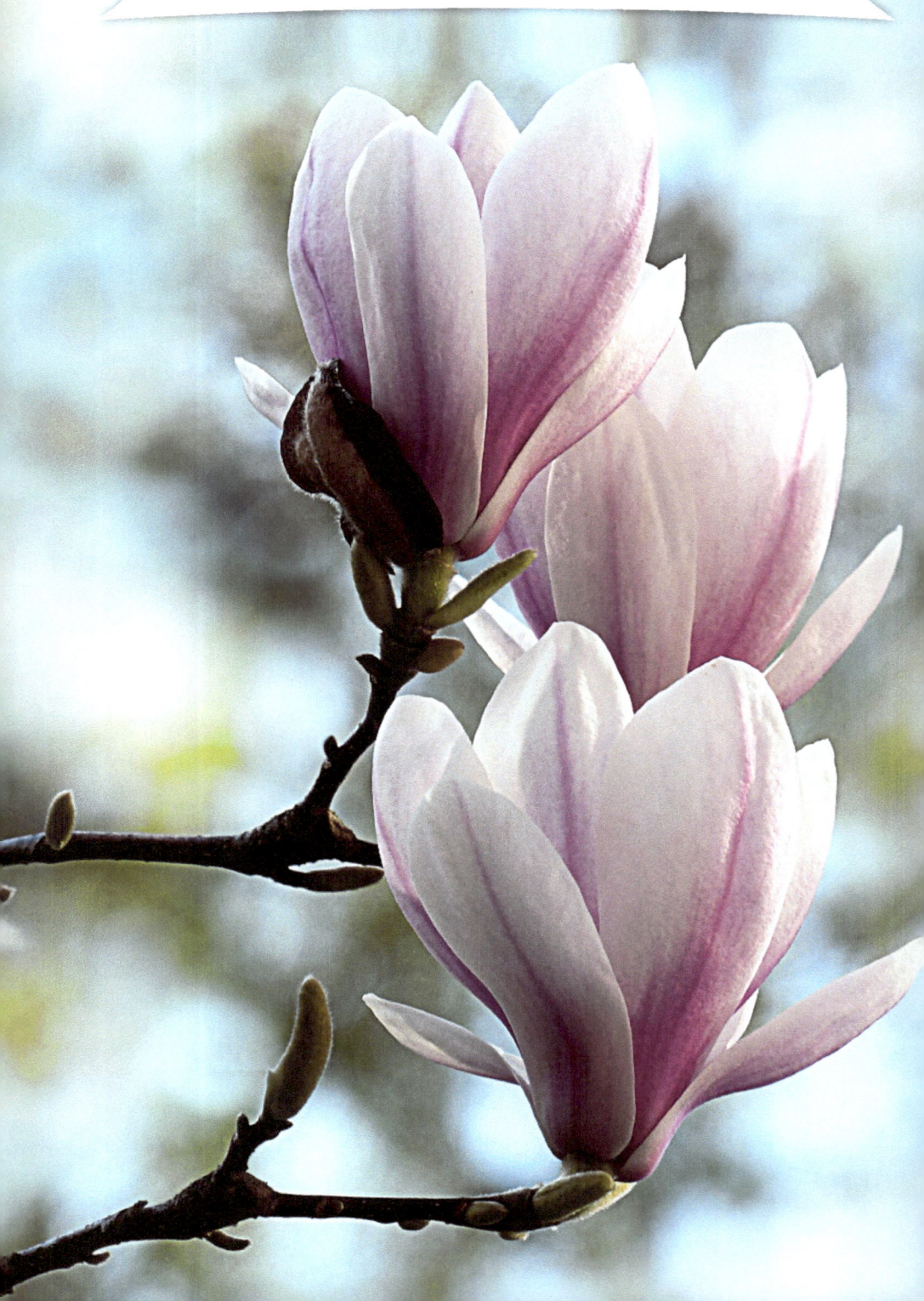

MAGNOLIA

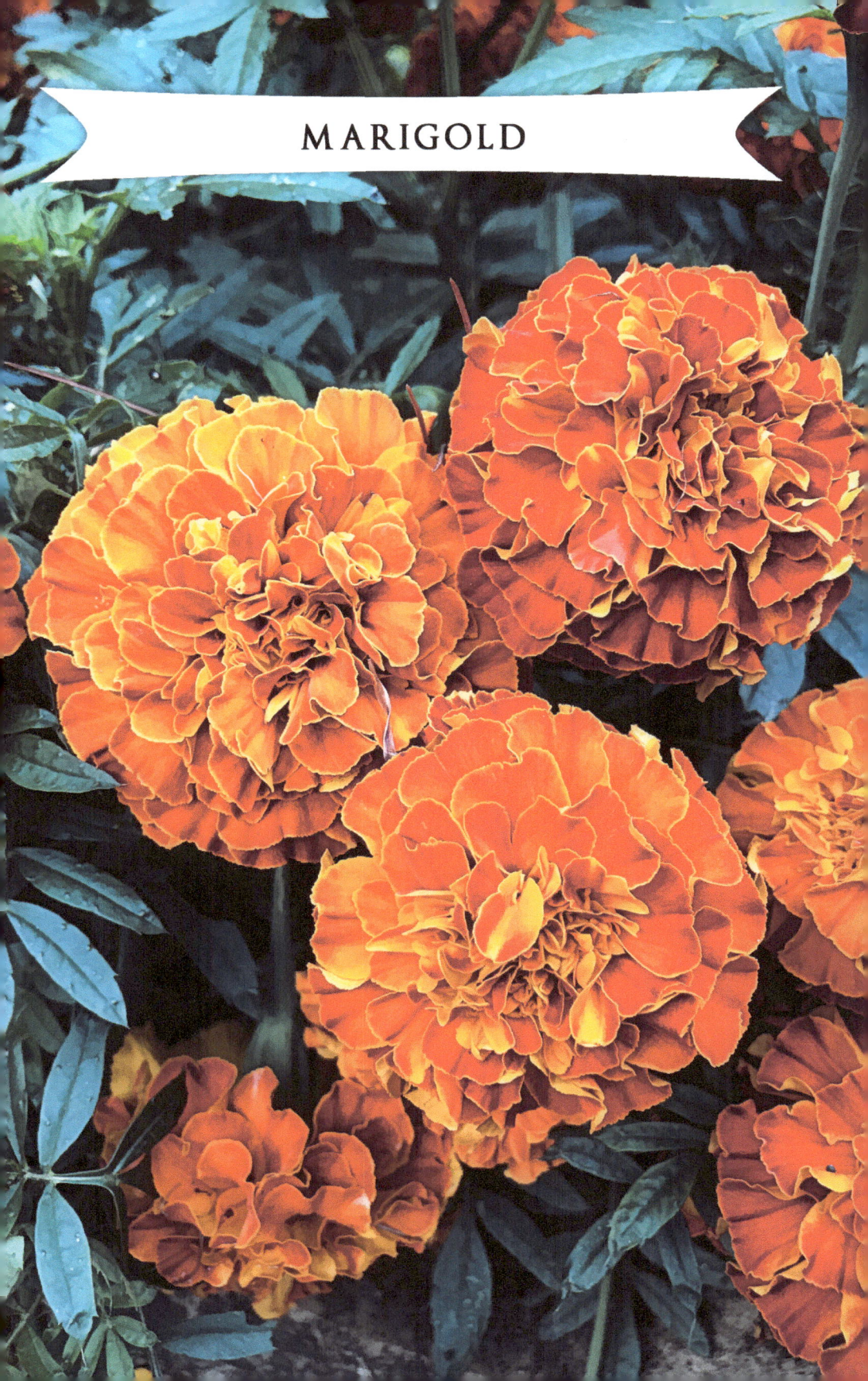

MARIGOLD

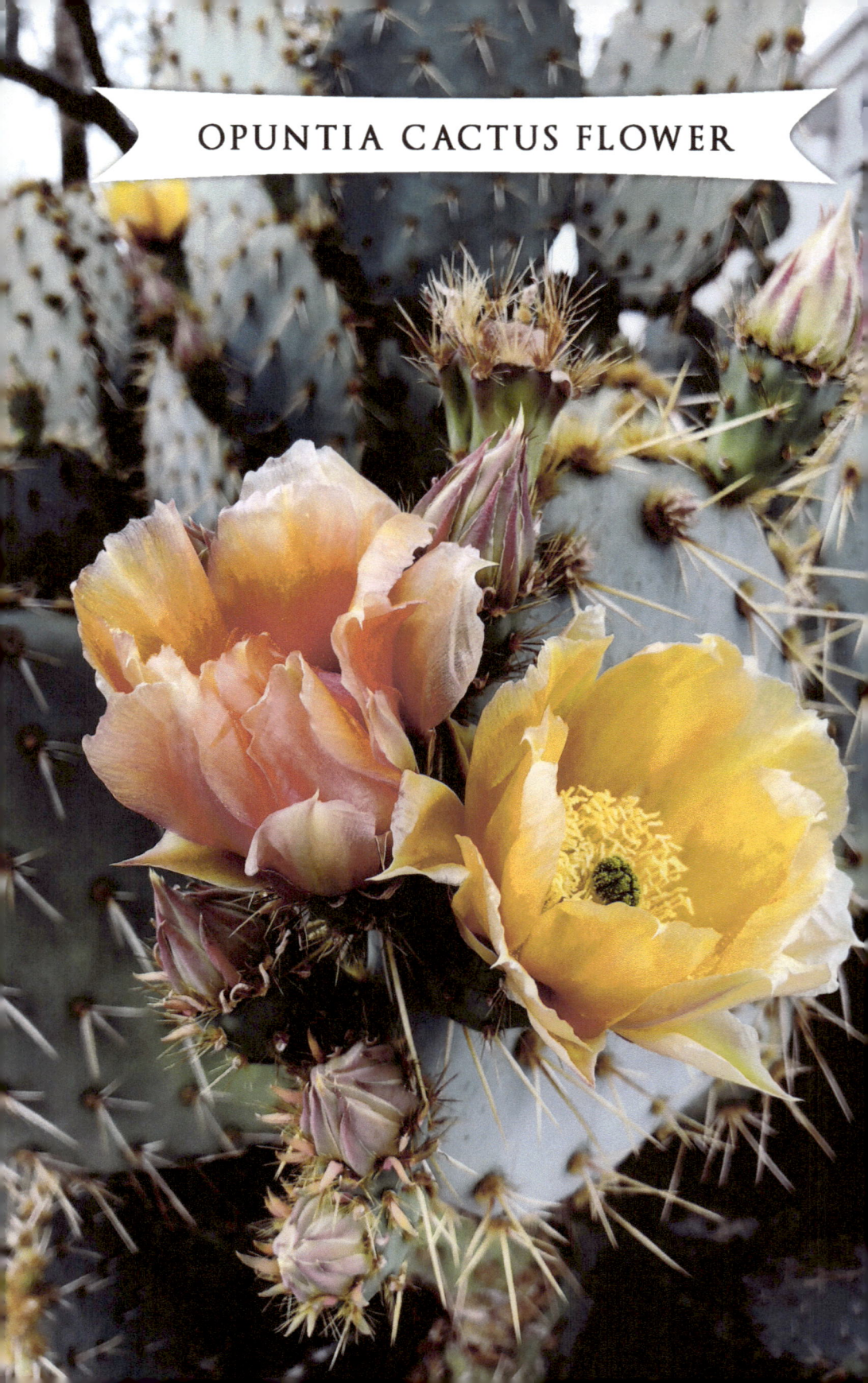

OPUNTIA CACTUS FLOWER

ORCHID

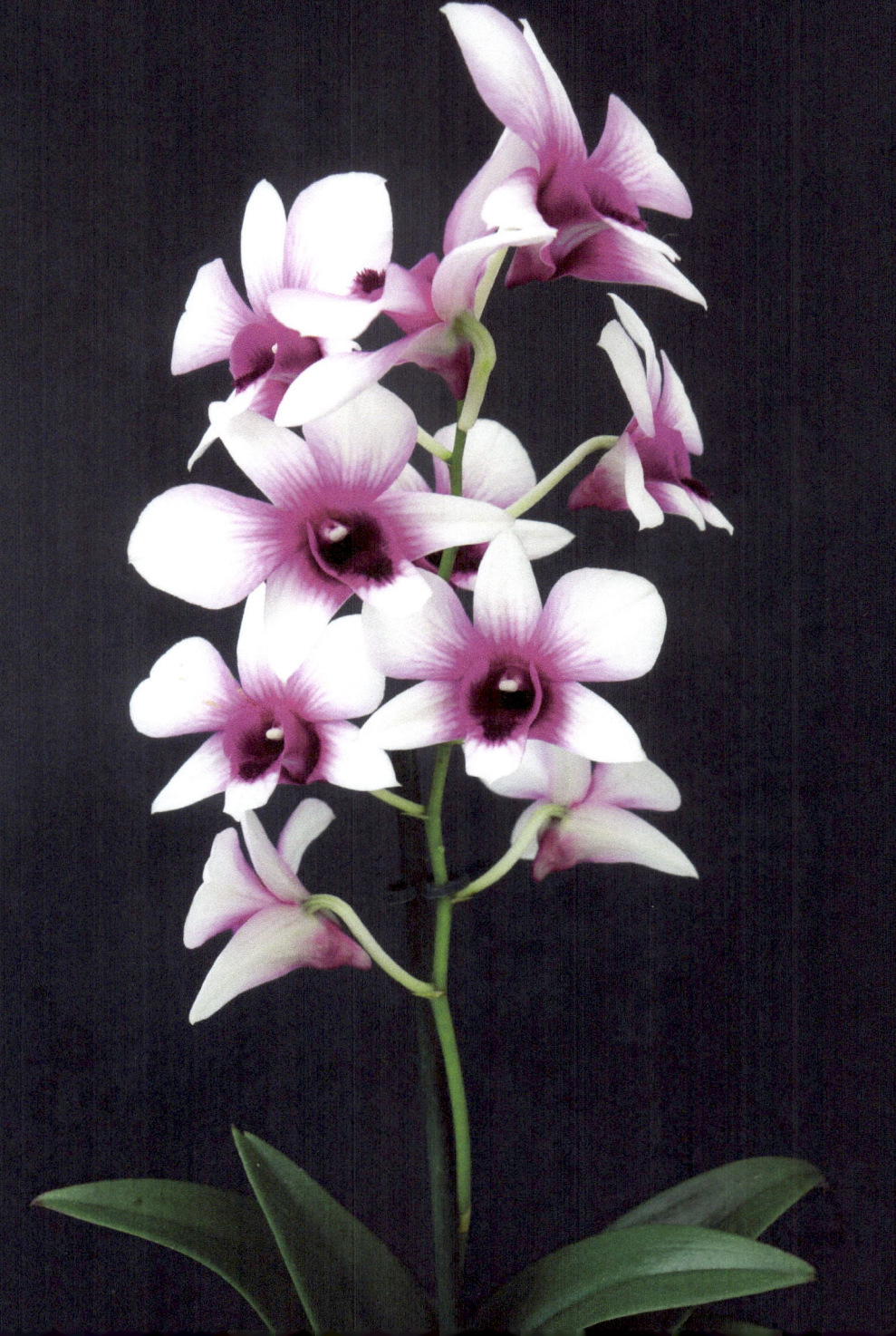

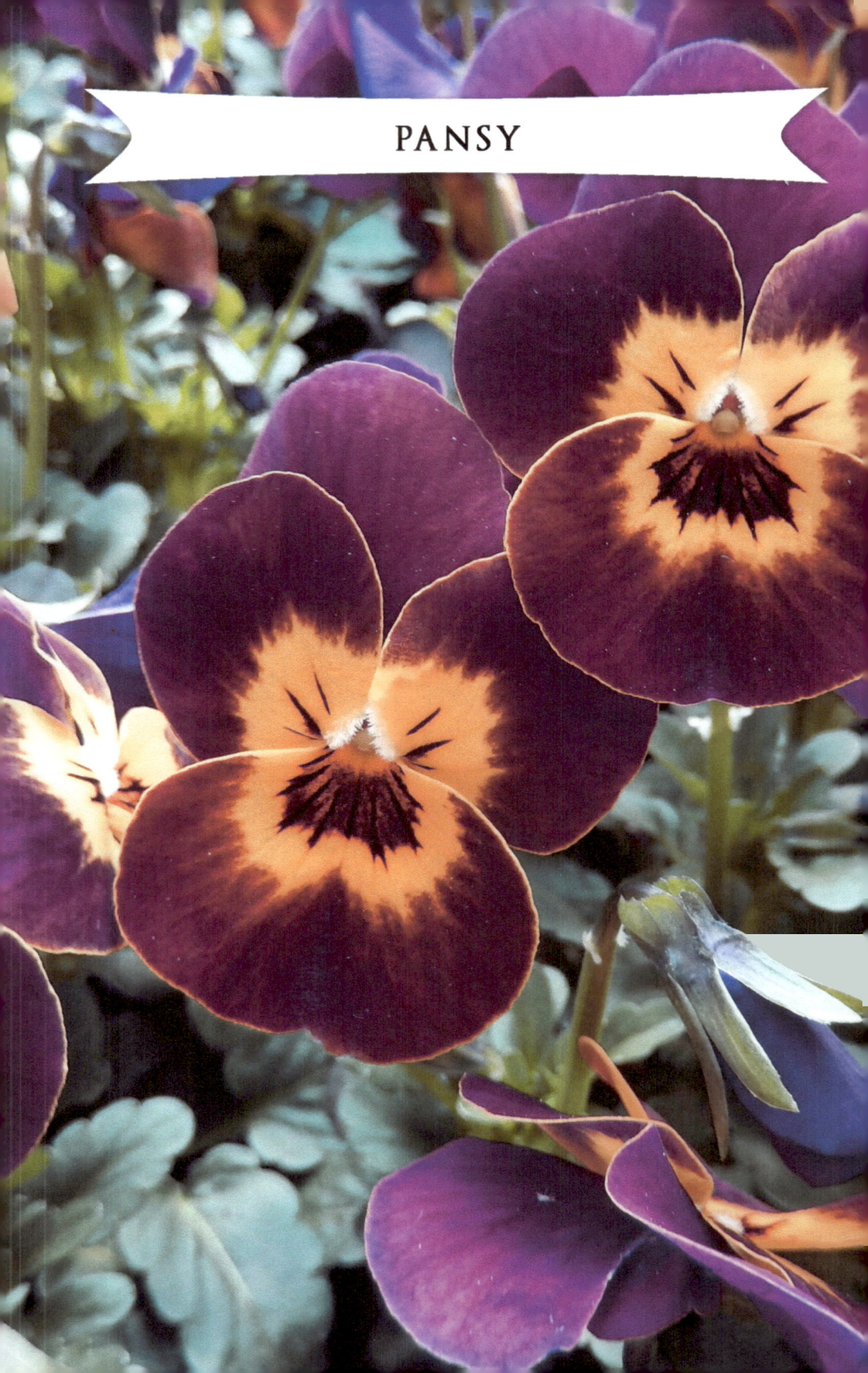

PANSY

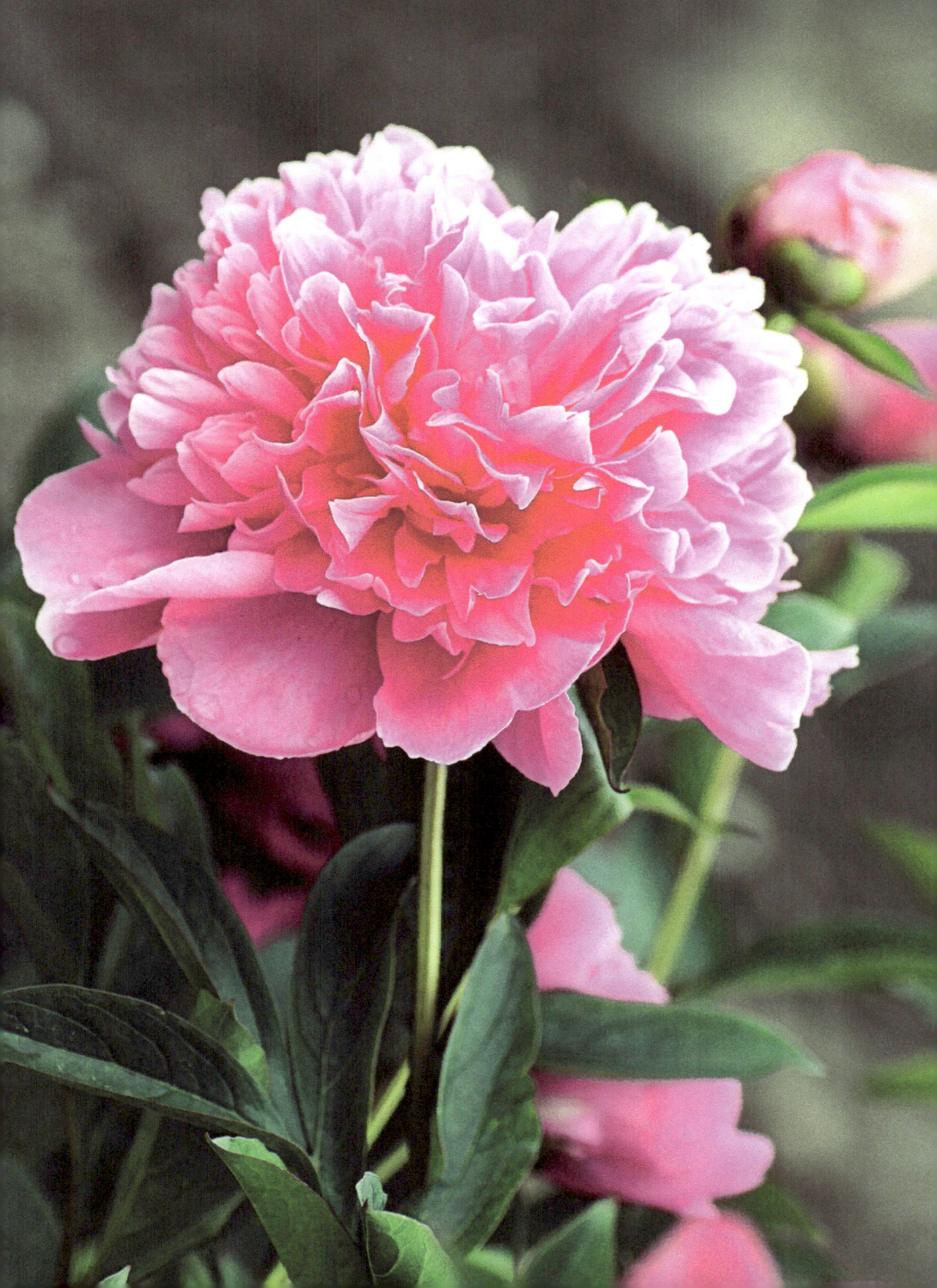

PEONY

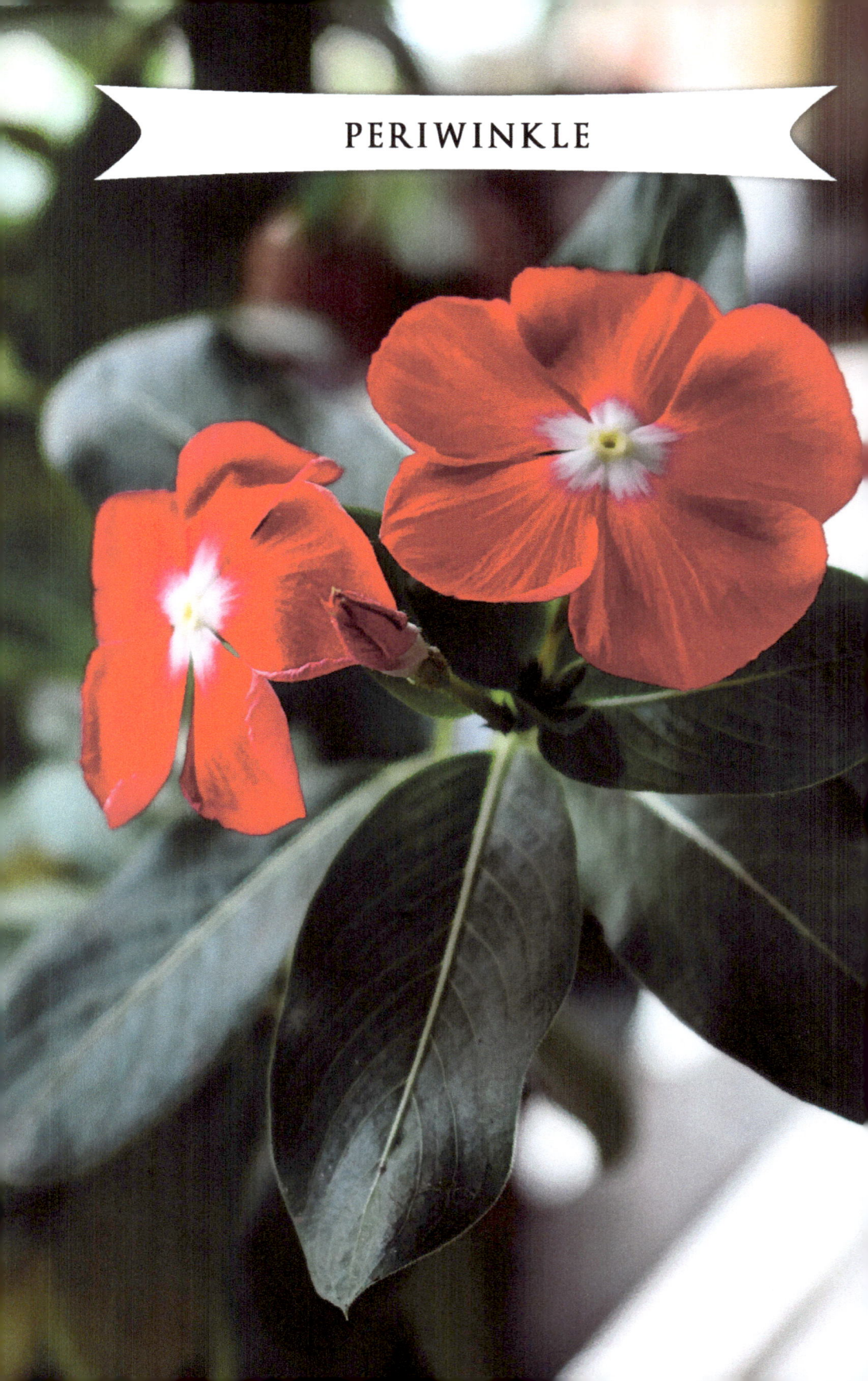

PERIWINKLE

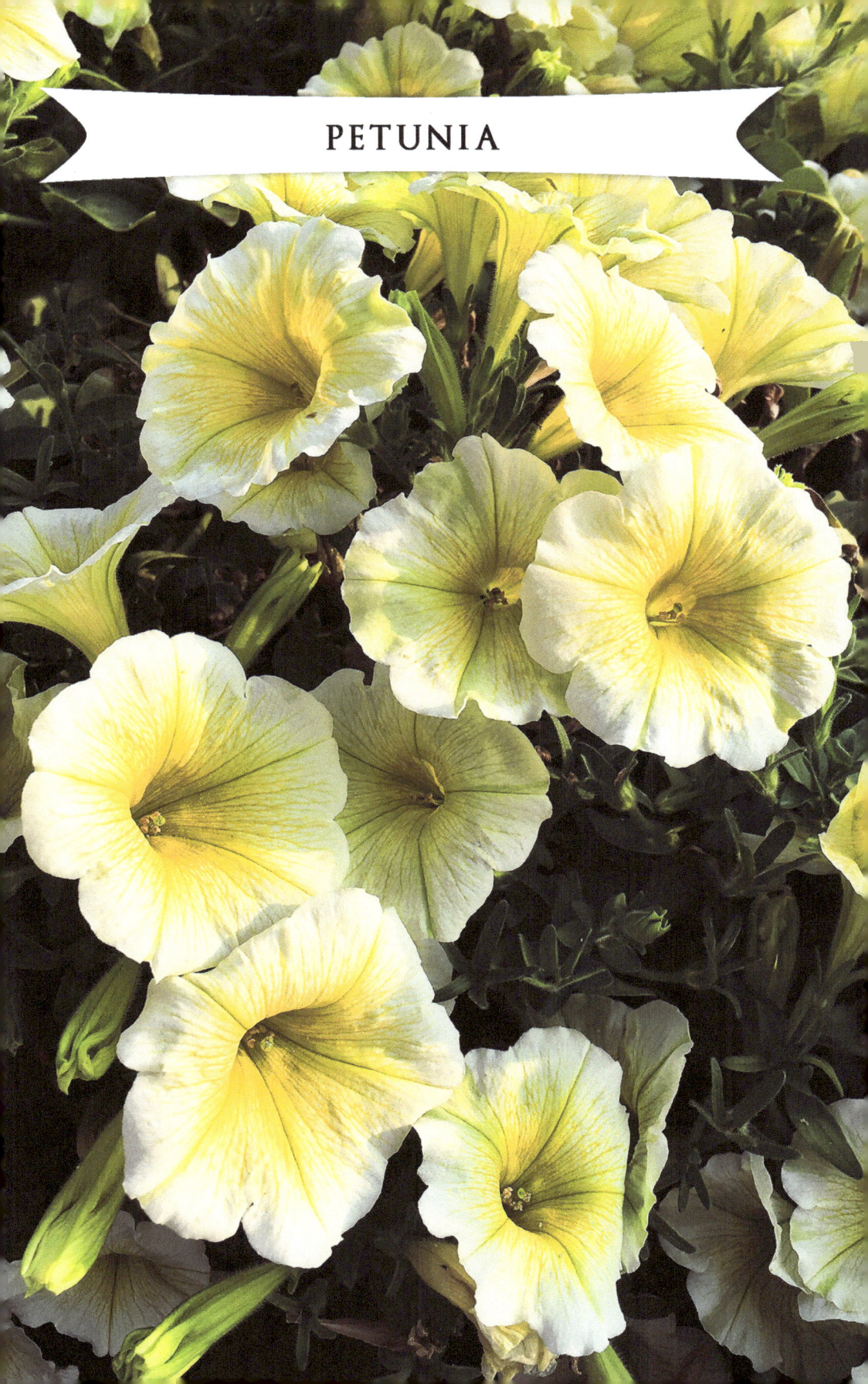

PETUNIA

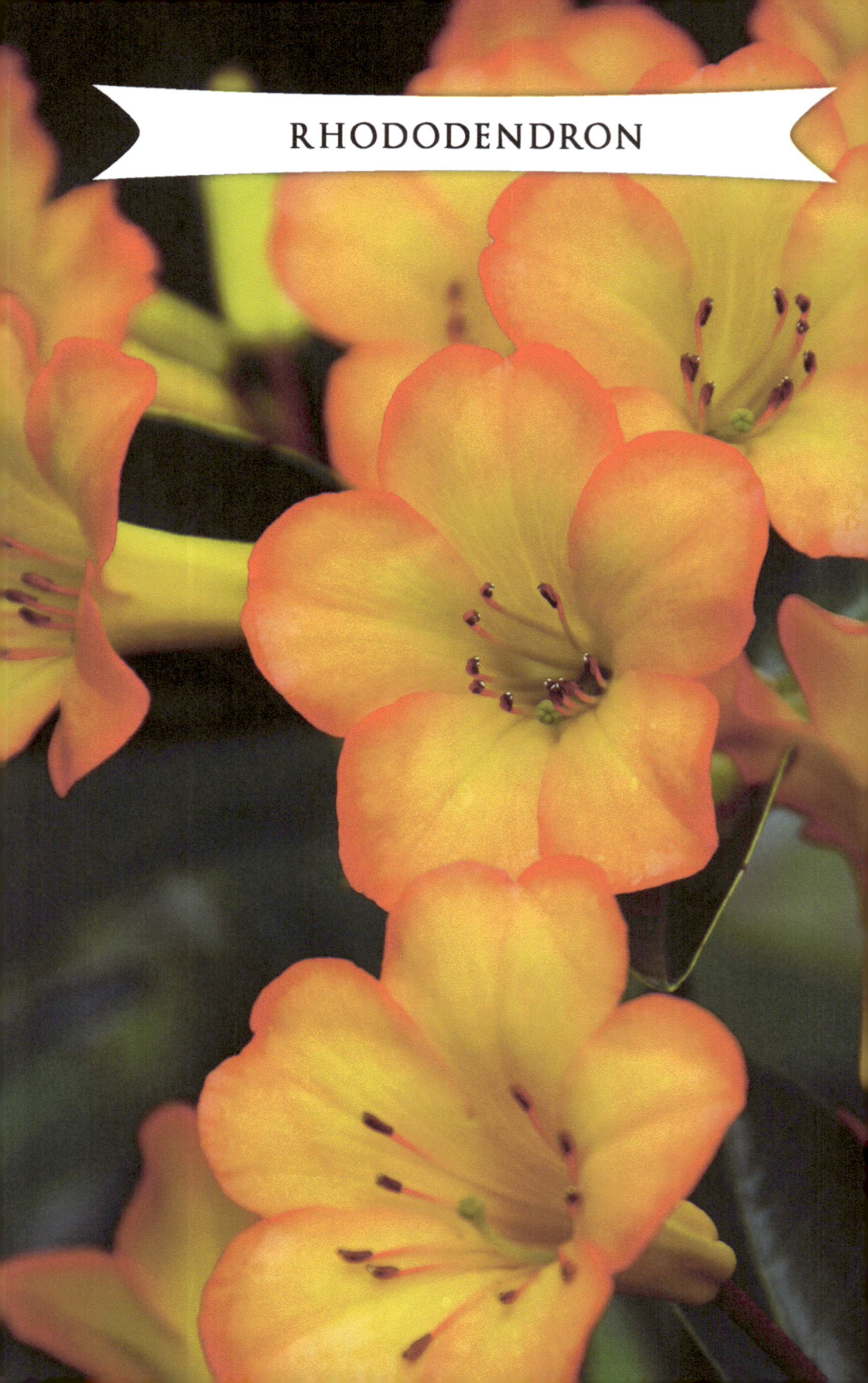

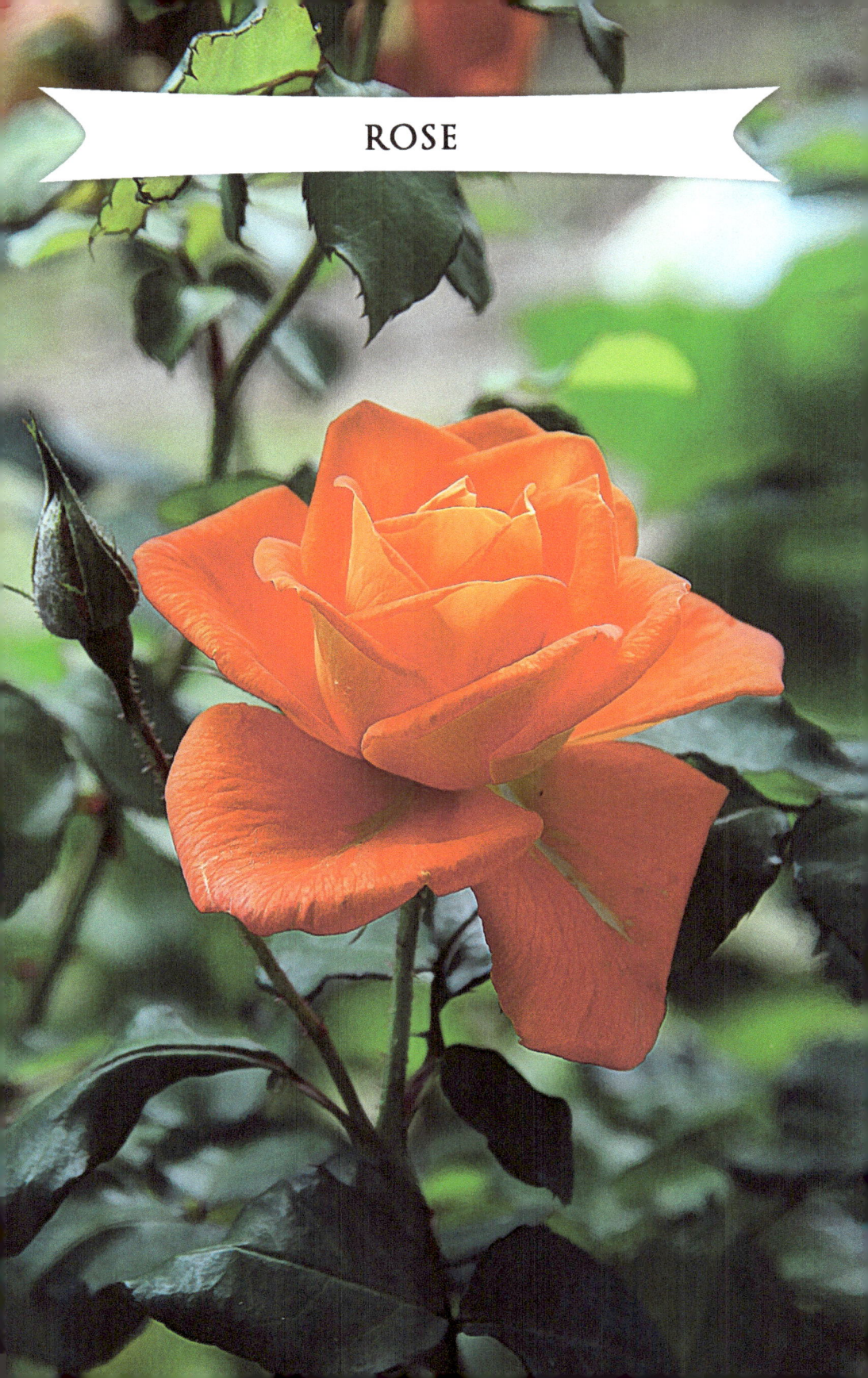

ROSE

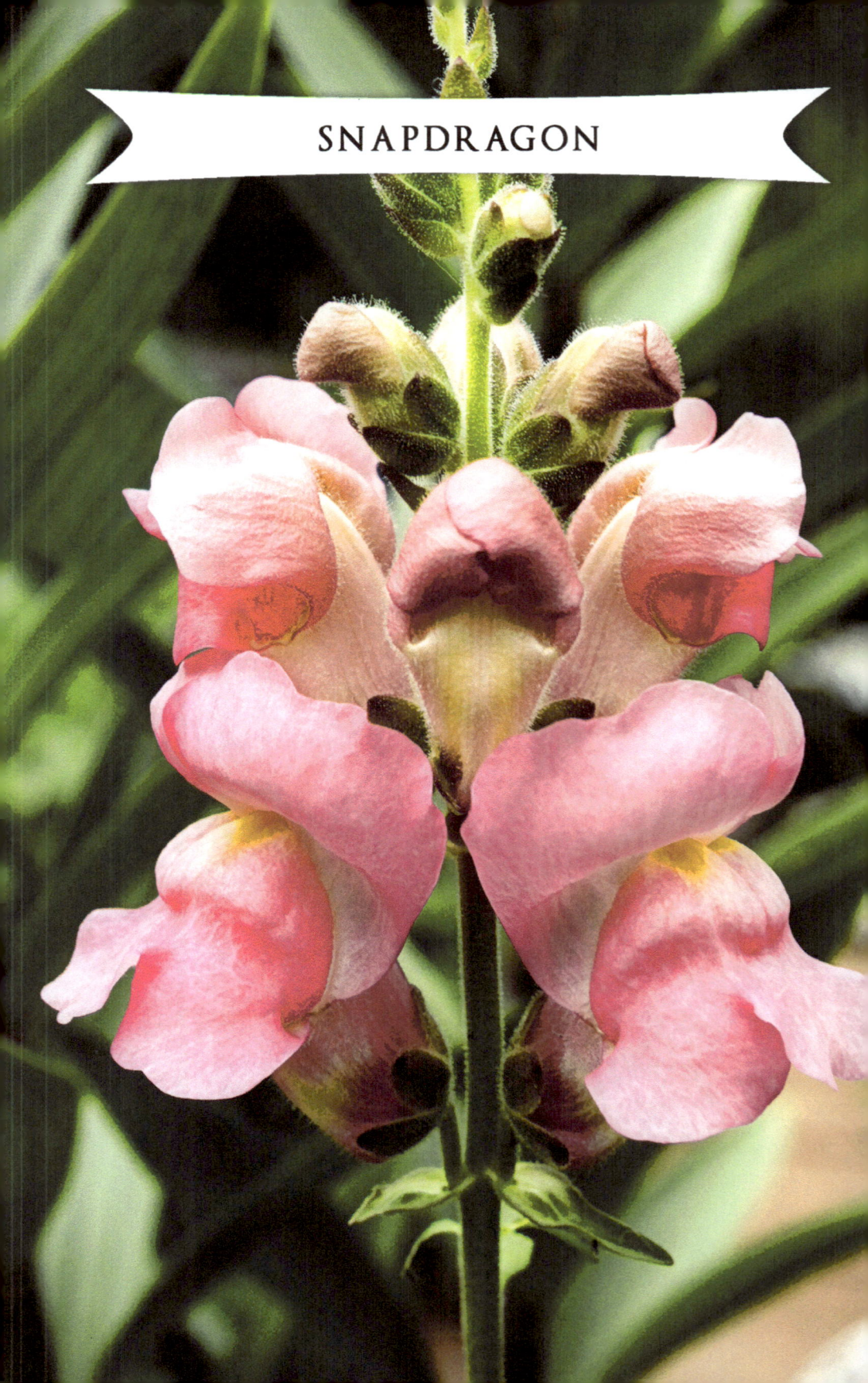

SNAPDRAGON

SNOWDROP

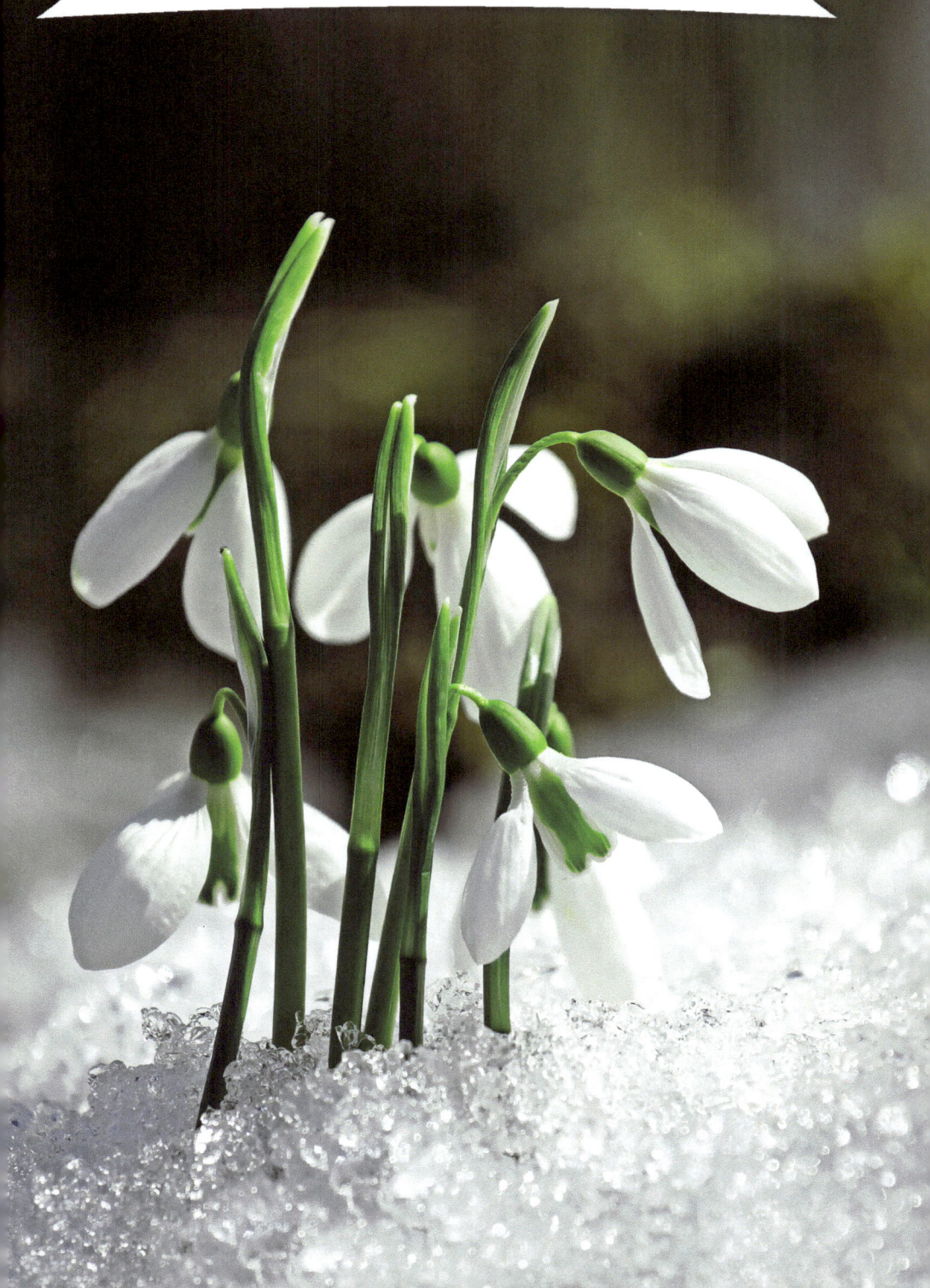

SUNFLOWER

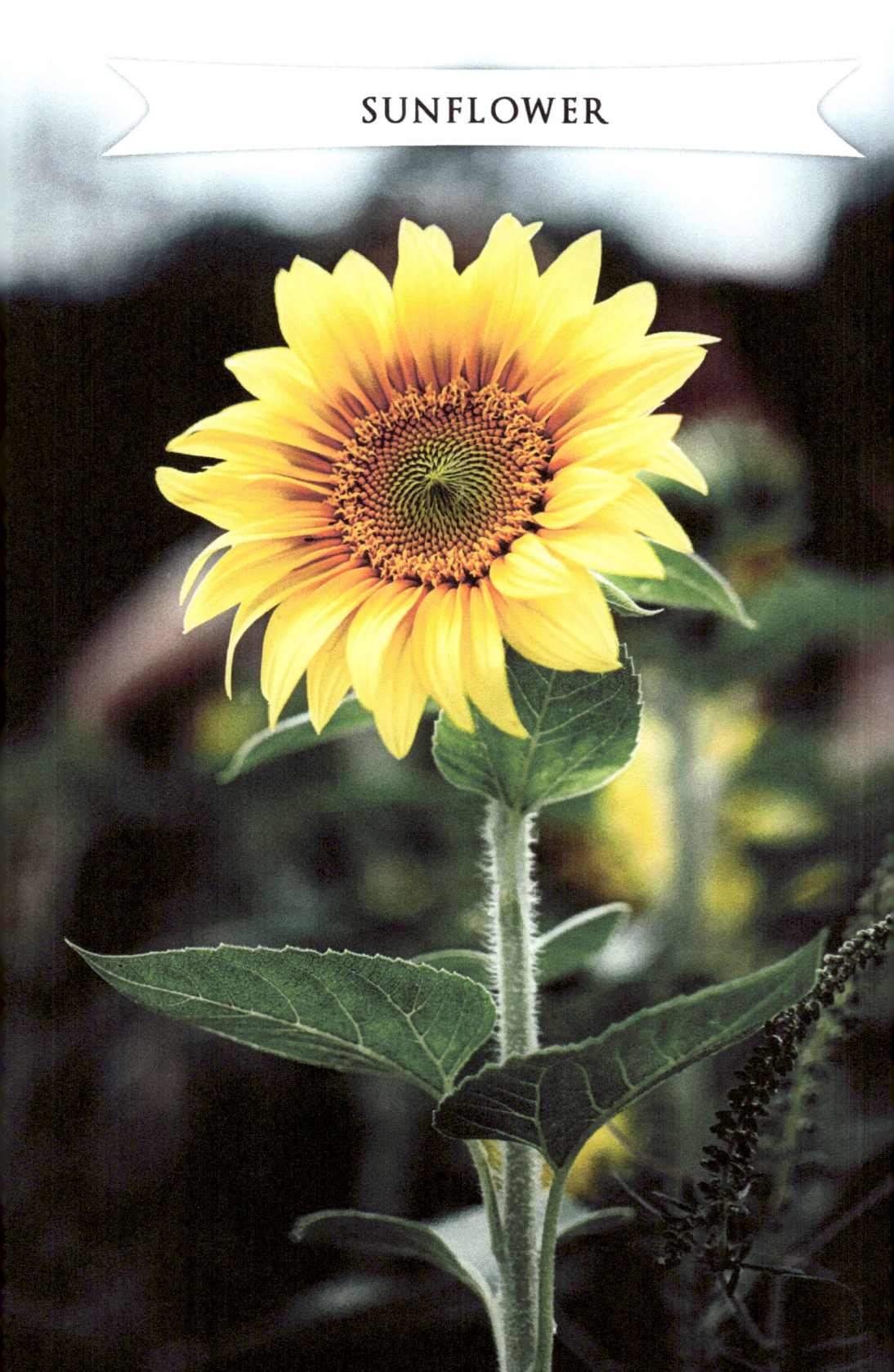

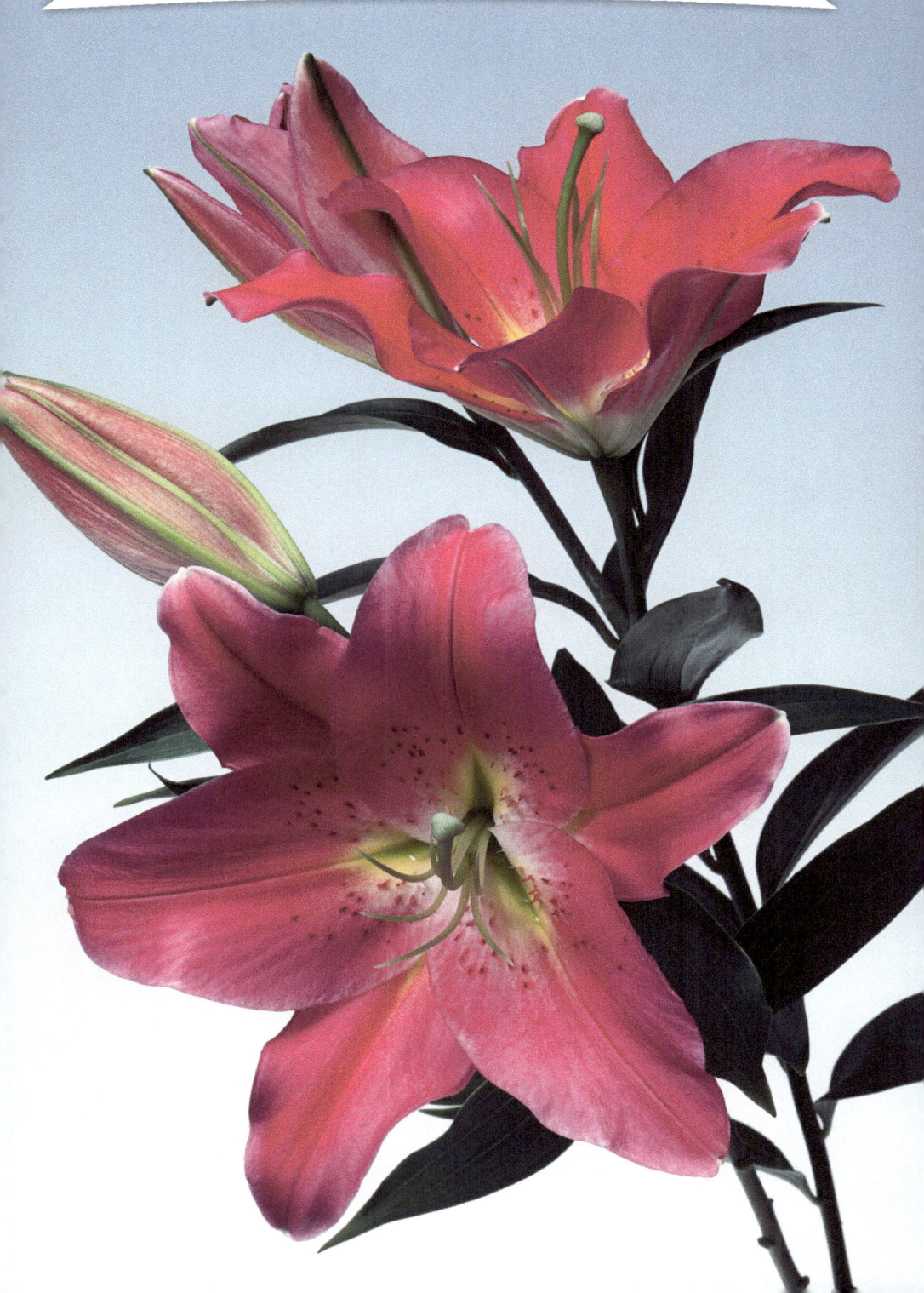

TIGER LILY

TULIP

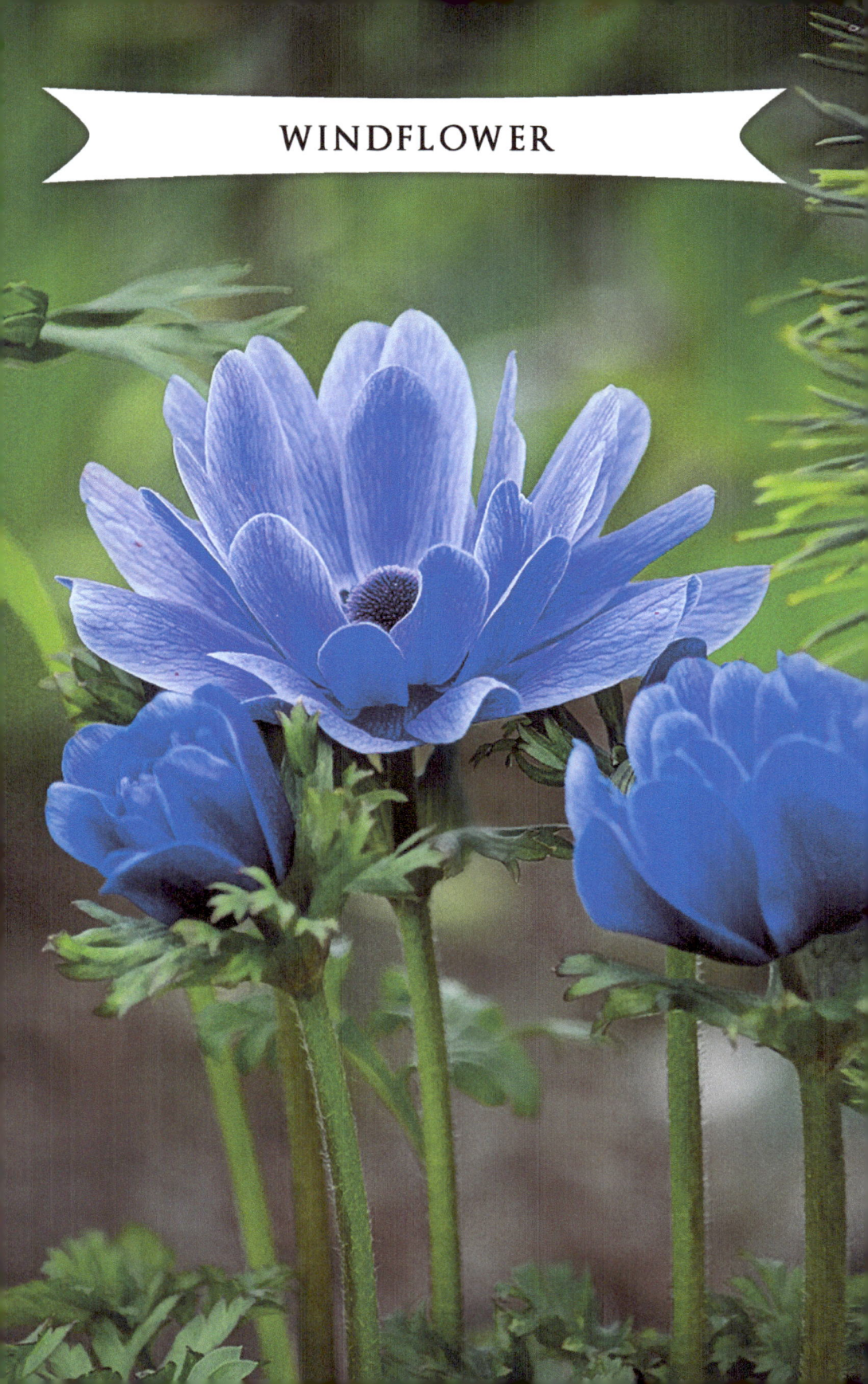

WINDFLOWER

www.ingramcontent.com/pod-product-compliance
Lightning Source LLC
Chambersburg PA
CBHW050757290526
45792CB00008B/2220